THE ANDROPAUSE MYSTERY

Unraveling truths about the
Male Menopause

ROBERT S. TAN, M.D.

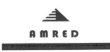

AMRED

AMRED Publishing, Houston, Texas

i

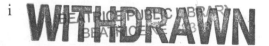

The Andropause Mystery -

Unraveling truths about the Male Menopause

AMRED Publishing is a Division of AMRED Consulting L.L.C., located at www.amred.com

Visit us on line at http://www.andropausemystery.com to order more copies, offer feedback and learn about the author's work.

ISBN 0-9707061-0-3

Disclaimer -

Manufactured in the United States of America

ACKNOWLEDGEMENTS

I was continuously supported and encouraged by my dear wife. Grace has taught me the precious lessons on perseverance and adaptation in life.

I am also deeply grateful to my patients for they have taught me so much about being a doctor.

I thank S.Z. Nasr M.D. for his kind contribution, insights and friendship and P. S. Philips M.D. for her invaluable help in the Andropause study.

We appreciate Larry & Cynthia Kirkpatrick who have given so much of themselves.

The support that was given by our parents and the extended family has permitted us to develop to our fullest.

Good friends and associates- I cannot mention them all, but each one is cherished.

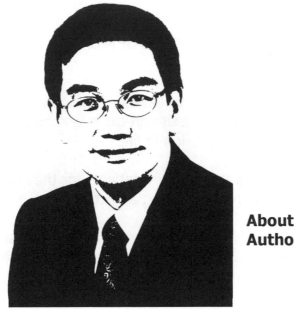

**About the
Author**

Dr. Robert Tan is a practicing physician specializing in Geriatric Medicine in Houston, Texas. As a Fellowship trained Board Certified physician with duties as a Medical Director, he spends his time attending to patients who suffer from Age related issues. He also teaches at the University of Texas and has extensively published scientific literature in several medical journals. He was elected a Fellow of the American Geriatrics Society and is nationally and internationally recognized for his pioneering research work on the Andropause.

Contents

Preface:
Why I got excited about the Andropause

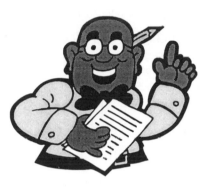

What they did not teach me in my medical training

During my extensive training as a physician, I was taught, among a myriad of other issues, how to recognize and treat the menopause. I learned that women had a cessation of menstrual periods and thereafter, they no longer were able to bear children. During this change of life, women were more likely to be depressed, started having osteoporosis and were at greater risk for events such as strokes and heart disease. Hormonal therapy with estrogens seems to be able to reverse, or at least reduce, some of these adverse situations. For several years, I questioned if men underwent a similar process. In the course of my clinical practice, I noticed that male patients experienced some of the events such as depression and bone loss, similar to post-menopausal women. Medical textbooks do not delineate the change of life as a male issue but focus mainly on women, and elaborate preventive measures primarily for the latter. However, data from research suggest that endocrine changes do occur in men as they age.

By training and clinical practice, I am a Geriatrician, specializing in Care of the Elderly. I realize that there are indeed some very similar events in older males, in terms of physiological, psychosocial and biochemical changes, as compared to older women. A series of clinical events challenged me to ponder whether men undergo hormonal changes similar to women. Let me narrate my encounter with a charming eighty five year old patient, who made an impact on my career and the way I currently think about my older male patient.

My eighty-five year old childless patient

Several years ago, I visited an elderly gentleman in a nursing home. This rather routine visit proved to be one of the turning points in my medical career. This patient had just broken his arm following minimal trauma and was there for a period of rehabilitation. His bones were so sensitive to pain that the mere act of being carried to the bathroom by the aides brought about excruciating pain in his arms. My first thought was perhaps a form of cancer had got to his bones and made them brittle and sensitive. When I examined him, he appeared tired, pale and lacked all vigor. Further examination revealed that his memory had deteriorated, his sexual organs were shrunken and he had no hair in his armpits or in his genital area. In fact, he claimed that he had not needed to shave for the past 20 years, which I thought was a great convenience! I had an accompanying resident, and explained to him that this was a case of testosterone deficiency – the patient was suffering from "hypogonadism". "Hypo" means low and "gonadism" refers to the gonads or testes. Sure enough, laboratory testing confirmed his hypogonadic state. Both his total as well as his free (unbound portion) of testosterone was low.

I decided to treat him with intramuscular testosterone injections given once every 2 weeks, after checking that his prostate was normal. At that time, although testosterone replacement for younger hypogonadic men was fairly established, testosterone replacement for older men was little heard of. I even had difficulty convincing the pharmacy to release the medication. After 3 months, he started growing a beard and began walking again. His fracture had healed and his memory actually improved. He started asking me if he could be discharged from the nursing home. Most importantly, he asked me if he could start a family - he was childless at this point. I jokingly discussed this with his eighty year-old wife, who persuaded me to keep him in the nursing home!

I had stumbled upon the potential of testosterone replacement in older men, something never taught to me before or much discussed in the medical literature. The alarming statistic is that about 25 - 35% of men over 65 may be hypogonadic! This works out to be close to 5 million men in America, which is almost an epidemic proportion. However, less than 5% of older men are treated for hypogonadism, so that the potential for improved quality of life for the older male is staggering.

New frontier

Shortly after my encounter with this 85 year-old patient, I decided to review the medical literature and found that there was surprisingly little research in the area of the male menopause or Andropause. Even on the internet, a search for "Andropause" at the time of writing in the National Institute of Health's "PubMed " site (http://www4.ncbi.nlm.nih.gov/PubMed/) retrieves very little clinical research in this topic, other than my research article posted there. Some review articles exist, but these basically summarize the research done by others and express an opinion. So far, the articles and books written on the Andropause are mostly based on personal anecdotal experiences. It is the purpose of this book to unravel truths and dispel myths.

One dictionary I referred to defined Andropause as "a time in life of the older male that is associated with a

reordering of life associated with low testosterone levels."
The Andropause is not to be confused with the "mid-life
crisis", which typically occurs earlier by one to two decades.
Some men undergo a mid life crisis, as if they do not want
to loose the youthful manhood they previously had. They
engage in activities more appropriate for younger years,
such as purchasing a sports car, wearing trendy clothes or
getting involved in extramarital affairs. The Andropause is
distinct as it is a physiological state rather than
a psychological state (as in the mid-life crisis). Also, I believe
that the Andropause is not a pathological or disease state
and it does happen to most men eventually, but not all men
in a uniform way. One of my areas of research is to find out
why it affects some men prematurely. What protects some
men from the Andropause, and why are some men more
susceptible? What are the risk factors for Andropause, and
how can we prevent it from occurring?

I was excited at the possibility of testosterone
replacement for older men and presented the case of the
childless elderly man in a nursing home at The American
Geriatrics Society. It did not receive very much attention as
it was mainly a case report and not a large scale randomized
controlled study, which seems today to be the gold standard
for investigative trials. In any event, several patients of mine
thereafter, who were beyond Andropause, were started on
testosterone replacement. While some reported success,
others did not. Some even exhibited hypersexuality, for
which testosterone had to be stopped!

Testosterone has been off patent for several decades and it was difficult to convince sources for funding, but I continued researching into this, often collecting data as I went about my busy clinical practice and teaching responsibilities. I was further inspired by the findings of other physician scientists working on testosterone replacement in Atlanta, St. Louis, Houston and Los Angeles. In Britain, an andrologist also reported interesting results in his private practice in Harley Street. The Emory University group found increase in muscle strength following replacing some older men with testosterone. The study was very well regarded but unfortunately lacked numbers and follow up was limited to less than 2 years. Despite this, the study attracted attention from the media such as Newsweek, CNN and CBS.

My own research work has focused on defining what Andropause means to older men. I was interested in their perceptions of this entity. In addition, I was interested in the epidemiological profiles of men who said they underwent the Andropause. I collected data on when the onset of Andropause was. I also questioned men on whether current medical treatments were adequate. Since Andropause can be considered part of the aging process in some males, I was also interested in identifying some of the risk factors. By identifying the risk factors, preventive measures could be introduced to males to delay the Andropause, just as for the menopause in females.

Recently, I have been excited about the possibility of using testosterone to improve memory in demented men who are at the same time hypogonadic. This work is ongoing at the moment, but I have preliminary results indicating a significant success rate. Unfortunately the improvement in cognition was short-lived, generally lasting about 6 months only, before starting to decline again. This will be explained in a later chapter, so hang on patiently until I spill the beans!

It is my hope that you will enjoy reading this book. Perhaps you are trying to find out a little of the changes that are occurring in you physiologically. Alternatively, you could be a spouse or a child of someone undergoing the changes associated with Andropause, someone you dearly love. You may be yearning for clarification and direction in the midst of bewildered confusion. My hope is that we now crusade for men what we crusaded for women undergoing the menopause 3 decades ago.

Chapter 1.
Andropause - Fact or fiction?

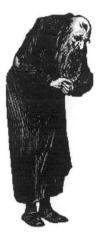

Growing Old

The aging process is associated with the loss of muscle mass, bone density, mental aptitude, multi-organ efficiency and general functionality, especially after the age of 40. Fat replaces muscle, and on average, males lose 12 to 15 pounds of muscle. Between the ages of 40 to 70 years, the average male also loses 15% of his bone mass and nearly 2 inches of his height, mainly as a result from osteoporosis. After age 40, even the testicles shrink and by age 70, 15% of men in this country are impotent. These alarming statistics are sad but true facts of the aging process.

The Andropause is the time in a man's life when the hormones naturally decline. Mosby's Medical Dictionary defines the Andropause as "a change of life for males that may be expressed in terms of a career change, divorce, or reordering of life. It is associated with a decline in androgen levels that occurs in men during their late forties or early fifties". Many have questioned whether the male menopause is more myth than reality. In truth there is an undeniable hormonal decline as one ages, and this in turn aggravates the aging process.

Nevertheless, some men are still able to father children in their eighties, a famous example being Charlie Chaplain, the great comedian. This may prove a point that the Andropause is not universal, occurring in some, but not all, men. The changes come about because of down regulation of hormones including testosterone. I will try to define hormones. Hormones are chemicals that are produced in the body by organs called endocrine glands, and they regulate the function of other organs. Although mainly natural, hormones can be artificially synthesized today. Some examples of hormones include insulin, which regulates blood sugar, thyroxine, which regulates overall metabolism, and estrogens, which regulate female functions including reproduction. Hormones in themselves are regulated by a feedback system. It is a hierarchal system of control with the hypothalamus and pituitary gland being control centers. Regulatory or trophic hormones in turn control the function of individual hormones.

Let us next discuss what symptoms men have in association with the Andropause.

What Symptoms are associated with the Andropause?

Four to 5 million men are hypogonadic in the United States, and 60% are over the age of 65. However, statistics reveal that only 5% are treated for symptoms related to the Andropause. Between the ages of 50 to 70, some men report symptoms such as erectile dysfunction (failure to achieve an erection), general tiredness, mood changes, night sweats and sometimes palpitations. From my own research, which will be described in detail in a later chapter, I found that most men attributed erectile dysfunction to be the most significant event of the Andropause for them. Obviously erectile dysfunction can have many other causes including psychogenic ones, and a fuller discussion will be undertaken in later chapters.

Apart from erectile dysfunction, mood changes can take place too. Some patients of mine have complained of nervousness, irritability and even depression. Other patients undergoing andropausal changes report the feelings of wanting to be closer to family and friends. Men often focus too intently on their career, money and power in their earlier life, often neglecting family and friends. In the andropausal years, men and take on a more "maternal" role, as if transitioning to become more motherly than fatherly. They

11

become more concerned about their friends and family, as if regretting their former attitudes. It is interesting that many patients do not sense these changes in themselves, but rather it is the spouse that notices this and tells me that he is undergoing "the menopause"!

In andropausal men, night sweats and palpitations occur because of an overactive autonomic system in response to falling testosterone levels. Overactivity of the autonomic system can occur in diabetic patients and it is important not to confuse symptoms of diabetic autonomic neuropathy with that of the Andropause. Some disease states like hyperhidrosis, viral and parasitic infections can cause excessive sweating. Obviously a humid night in the tropics without air conditioning does the same, even for normal individuals!

It is important not to dismiss or misdiagnose physiological changes related to the Andropause. At the same time, it is important not to over label the Andropause and miss some important pathology, like malaria for instance!

Are there Signs associated with the Andropause?

Symptoms are what patients feel, signs are what is observed by the clinician. For example, dizziness is a symptom and blood pressure is a sign. So, are there signs of the Andropause that could be picked up by a clinician or a significant other who has noticed the changes? The answer is yes, and these are summarized below.

Signs & Symptoms of Hypogonadism that occur in the Andropause

---

1. Loss of hair in the armpits and axilla
2. Testicles become smaller in size
3. Decreased Libido or low sex drive
4. Erectile Dysfunction or impotence
5. Lethargy or tiredness
6. Depression
7. Decreased muscle strength
8. Oligospermia or low sperm count
9. Decrease bone density

Androgens basically create "masculinity" and the loss of androgens such as testosterone leads to physical changes. Women in their post-menopausal years complain of dryness in their vagina, skin and sometimes even a lowering of the pitch of voice. The dryness in the vagina could result in dyspareunia or pain on intercourse. In men, subtle changes occur in the post-andropausal years. The once dashing Valentino looks are now exchanged for something much less eye-catching. Hardened muscle disappears and instead, flabby fat accumulates as one gets older. This distorts the physique from an athletic "android" to one with a beer belly and little muscle. The skin also gets dry, and there is hair loss. Hair loss occurs not only in the scalp, but also in the genital area as well as in the axilla. The testes also atrophy (get smaller) slowly. There is loss of height because of osteoporosis and the spine gets curved from wedge compression fractures. It is important to realize that testosterone can maintain bone integrity just like estrogens in women.

Psychological challenges older males face in the Andropause

Throughout the life of a male there are several psychological issues that he struggles with, and these challenges are often amplified during the time of the Andropause: -

1. His sexuality
2. His emotions
3. His mind
4. His courage
5. His productivity
6. His personality
7. His character
8. His boyish behaviors

The sexuality of a youthful man aged between 15 to 30 years when his testosterone was at an all time high, drops to the ebb during the Andropause. Young men often have testosterone levels exceeding 1000ng/dl. Compare this with 80 year-old men, whose average testosterone is 200ng/dl.

You might say the sexuality of a man in the Andropause is down 80%, a seemingly disastrous event.

I have noticed that older men tend to be closer to their family and are more interested in domestic issues than when they were younger. It is as if the lack of testosterone makes them more "feminine". They take on more homely roles of cooking, cleaning and looking after children. More often than not, they devote much more time and attention to their grandchildren than they had previously to their own children when they were parents themselves. Perhaps it is because they have more time during the andropausal years as they have probably retired by then. They usually also have more disposable income, having saved most of their lives, and are more willing to enjoy little pleasures around them, stopping to smell the roses. Their emotions become less "fiery" and take on a gentler aspect, so in a sense, the decline of testosterone enhances domestication skills.

In the andropausal years the mind becomes less sharp and nimble. The older male becomes less swift in mental calculations and his judgment is not as accurate as before. Perhaps he used to make razor-sharp business deals, but now he makes blatant mistakes and incurs painful financial losses. Oftentimes, he attributes it to aging, but in truth it may be partly due to the decline of testosterone. In more severe cases, the memory gets impaired too, and with time, dementia may even set in.

Although once willing to take risks of all sorts, the andropausal man becomes more conservative and fears treading in unclear waters. They no longer participate in roller coasters and bungee jumping, but rather watch these on TV instead. Most loose courage to take on new ventures and feel it is a time to retire and to "take it easy". However, fear and courage take on a different perspective in the andropausal years, especially in the older age group of the eighties and nineties. A study on fear was done whereby two groups of people were asked what they feared most. The younger group in the twenties said "death", but death was not what the eighty year olds feared most. It was their loss of independence. It is almost as if the elderly chide, "Death, where is thy sting?"

Productivity is at the core of a man's being. He feels happy when he creates something and is being noticed for it. He wants to feel contributory to his family and society. All his life he struggles to be the breadwinner for the family, and to get recognition at work for his efforts. In the days of early man, hunting and providing for his family and society was at the hub of function. For modern man, there may not be a need for barbaric hunting, but the board room still makes the same demands on his skills and abilities, and managing those complex business deals is akin to modern hunting. Andropause is a time of decline, when he is no longer as productive as he was before. Often he makes even less money than when he was younger, and feels threatened by younger more aggressive males biting into his turf.

A man's personality may not stay the same over the years of his life. In younger days the fiery younger male is impulsive, intolerant and ambitious. With the passage of time, various experiences and the fall in testosterone, quite a different male may emerge in later years. The red hot male often converts to a mellow yellow version, becoming more "feminine" and "domesticated", and taking on less challenges in the outside world, often preferring the cozy security of family and close friends. He is much less active, prefers his couch to watch television, and becomes weaker from lack of exercise.

Deep inside every man is the desire to remain young and be that little boy that he once was. This may become more marked after retirement as usually there is more spare time at hand. The andropausal man may relive his childhood days, often to the amazement of his partner or spouse! The mischief may be an extramarital affair, a new red sports car, a sudden passion for toy train sets, riding a bicycle, which he hadn't done for years, and so on. Sometimes of these childish acts may even be mistaken for Alzheimer's dementia!

Mr. A - a case of TB?

Mr. A, who was 55 years old, came to see me for night sweats. He was an executive in an oil exploration company and had noticed night sweats for about 2 months. He was smoking excessively too. He had traveled to South America for business, and was worried that he may have caught malaria or Tuberculosis (TB). He also had lost about 5 pounds in the past six months. Fortunately, he also mentioned to me that he had been under a lot of stress recently and "was having a problem with his down there", so much so that his wife wanted me to check him over. After the routine questions and examination, I proceeded to do some blood tests, ordered a TB skin test and a Chest X Ray. All the results came back indicating he was negative for TB. At the same time, because he had complained of erectile dysfunction, I measured his total testosterone level as well as his PSA. He had a total testosterone level of 120, which is about 30% of what he should be having at his age. As his prostate examination and his PSA were normal, I proceeded to treat him with intramuscular testosterone 200mg every 2 weeks, whilst reassuring him that he did not have TB. He was also advised to quit smoking. At follow up 3 months later, he was a dramatically changed person. He had put on some weight, which he boasted was muscle rather than fat, and he reported his erectile dysfunction had improved. Interestingly, he claimed his stress level was no different than before, but that he was coping better. He was also greatly relieved at not having the dreaded infectious diseases that he had feared.

Mr. B - Depression it was Not

I have spent several years researching depression in the elderly. It is a fascinating subject that is still evolving, and as yet, no one treatment seems to be effective all the time. Sometimes, medications such as antidepressants work well. At other times, it is psychotherapy that is effective. Even within the realm of antidepressants alone, there are several different classes of drugs. These include tricyclics (such as Elavil) and selective serotonin uptake inhibitors, commonly known as SSRIs (such as Prozac and Zoloft). Doses of antidepressants also vary with the age of the patient, and the older patient generally requires lower dosages.

Mr. B, a 70 year old nursing home resident had been treated with a SSRI antidepressant for several years. When I first encountered him, he was still profoundly depressed despite long-term treatment, and appeared lethargic. His functionality was failing and his mobility limited. In fact he was dependent on a walker. His memory was also questionable. A blood test revealed that his total testosterone was low at 180 ng/dl. Hence he began treatment with a course of intramuscular testosterone 200mg every 2 weeks. Amazingly, his moods improved, and he was taken off the antidepressant. If anything, the antidepressants were contributing to his erectile dysfunction. Some antidepressants cause impotence as a side effect. What was most remarkable to me was that he started to regain strength in his legs, and soon was walking without his walker! Testosterone is known to improve muscle strength as evidenced by the work of Dr. Tenover in Atlanta. Not only did Mr. B improve in his moods, he also regained substantial functional independence as a result of the therapy. This is another success story of testosterone replacement in a post-andropausal man.

Early scientific proof of the Andropause

The Andropause is likely to have existed since the creation of men. However, following advancements in public health in the last century, life expectancy generally increased, and men began to live into the sixties and seventies. As such, more scientists began to probe the existence of the Andropause. Arguably, the first scientific analysis of the Andropause was performed in the 1940's, in the midst of the Second World War. Dr. R J Douglas wrote on the diagnosis and treatment of the Andropause in the March 1941 issue of the Journal of Urology. This was followed by an editorial in the February 1942 issue of the Journal of the American Medical Association (JAMA). However, the landmark study delineating the male menopause was performed by Drs. Carl Heller and Gordon Myers at the Wayne University College of Medicine in Detroit. This was published in the October 21, 1944 issue of JAMA. Despite the turmoil of the war years, this article nevertheless received a lot of attention, including an editorial in the same journal. Reader's Digest also carried a similar article that very year.

In the study by Drs. Heller and Myers, all 23 male patients who demonstrated Andropause changes had markedly elevated FSH blood levels, comparable to castrated men. They thus established the first scientific proof that the Andropause was a reality. In 8 of the 23 cases, there was also evidence of testicular atrophy and degeneration by histology. The authors concluded that the male climacteric was different from that of psychoneurosis and psychogenic impotence. They also found that an intramuscular injection of testosterone proprionate reversed symptoms, but that oral and sublingual testosterone did not work. It was the opinion of these 2 doctors that although the male climacteric may occur as early as the third decade, it was a relatively rare syndrome and affected only a small proportion of men.

Perhaps that was the prevailing situation in the 1940's. My own study in the late 90's of 302 men revealed that almost 30% of men actually experienced andropause symptoms. Maybe, there is more openness today and a frankness that was not acceptable in those war years. However, I must state that the population I studied was people who had some health problem, and may have been exposed to huge amounts of tobacco. These additional factors could have contributed to the higher incidence as compared to that reported in the 1940's.

Menopause versus Andropause

Currently, the menopause is well defined. Women around the age of 50 years start developing hot flashes, palpitations and mood changes, symptoms of the pre-menopausal state. Their menstrual periods also become increasingly irregular, and eventually when the menses completely terminate, they cross the threshold of the Menopause. Although the menopause has existed since the creation of woman, it was not well understood until the twentieth century. At that time, advances in laboratory medicine allowed us to understand the hormonal effects associated with the menopause. From my own research, I have found that some men develop symptoms similar to pre-menopausal women. I would like to call this the pre-andropausal stage. I have used the words "some men" as this is not a universal event. Thirty percent of the elderly men I surveyed admitted to undergoing a male equivalent of menopause. This figure could obviously differ from region to region and could also be culturally biased. It is my observation that the andropause is more likely to be reported in cultures that are more open. In any event, the symptoms that men in my study described included erectile dysfunction, general weakness or fatigue, memory loss, intimacy issues and excessive night sweats. A small proportion of them complained about hot flashes and palpitations.

Unlike women, men do not experience a discrete physiological event such as the termination of the menses. Having said that, some men feel that the failure to have an erection is the equivalent of the end of menses. This is interesting as both events signal the end of a reproductive life. Overall, the symptoms of Andropause are more spread out over a longer period, in contradistinction to the menopause, which occurs generally over several months or at most a year.

Research has shown that there is a biochemical basis to this difference of timing. The cessation of the menses in women is associated with a dramatic decline in estrogen levels. Lowering of the estrogen levels leads to a compensatory rise of 2 hormones- Follicular Stimulating

Hormone (FSH) & Luteinizing Hormone (LH). This is an attempt by the pituitary gland in the brain to give the ovaries the last chance to produce more estrogens. FSH and LH are what we call regulatory hormones. This phenomenon is often described as the pituitary feedback system. In aging men, the decline of testosterone level leads to rises in the FSH and LH levels. The resultant high levels of FSH and LH act on the testes and the adrenals in attempt to produce more testosterone. However, in men the rise in FSH and LH levels is much less dramatic compared to women, as if there was some "protective effect". Why this is so, and why the andropause is of a much more gradual onset is unclear. In fact the gradual decline in testosterone in older men gradually has led to some clinicians calling the Andropause the "Androgen Decline in Aging Men" or ADAM syndrome. This, I feel is a more appropriate description of the natural event in men regarding testosterone decline with age. However, the decline is not exclusive to androgens alone, as other hormones such as Growth Hormone also do diminish with age.

The Andropause story is related to lowered levels of testosterone. However, what makes it more intriguing is that not all men who undergo andropausal symptoms actually have lowered testosterone levels. In my experience, the majority does, but not all. A normal testosterone level can also be associated with andropausal symptoms. This makes it frustrating as testosterone, although a useful treatment, may not work so effectively for symptoms such as erectile dysfunction when testosterone levels are adequate. Other hormones such as growth hormone, melatonin and endorphins are also lowered in the andropausal years, and may account for some of the changes in the andropause. Diabetes, often called the "mimic of all diseases" can lead to symptoms akin to Andropause. For instance, diabetics can develop complications such as autonomic neuropathy. In this condition the diabetic process destroys the small blood vessels that supply the autonomic nerves. This can lead to symptoms such as erectile dysfunction, night sweats, palpitations and so on, similarly experienced by patients undergoing Andropause. Thus it is important for diabetics to be treated appropriately, as appropriate management of diabetes may easily reverse some of the symptoms attributed to Andropause.

Testosterone levels decline with age, with the lowest level seen in men over 70 years. The age-related decline in testosterone secretion occurs at both control sites: the central (pituitary) and peripheral (testes). With aging there is also a rise in sex hormone binding globulin (SHBG), as well as a loss of the circadian (day versus night) rhythm of testosterone secretion. The phenomenon of the rise in SHBG with aging can be regarded as an adverse event. With more SHBG around, more testosterone wind up as being protein-bound, and less as free bioactive testosterone. Remember it is the free bioactive testosterone that is responsible for maintaining sexual and growth function in men. The younger male has testosterone levels that vary with the time of day, this helps the younger male adapt to events related to stress. However, in older men, the loss of the circadian rhythm results in the inability of older men to cope with stressor events. This has implication for the delivery system of testosterone replacement. Testosterone administered by a skin patch or a gel, called the transdermal form, is even more favorable than injections, because absorption through the skin is more gradual and less erratic.

A prominent researcher in the field of Andropause is Dr. Vermuelen from Belgium. He reported in one of his studies that plasma testosterone levels are below normal (defined as 250ng/dl) in only 7% of men between the ages of 40 to 60. However, 20% of men between the ages of 60 to 80 have below normal levels, and above 80 years, 35% have levels below normal. There could be several factors that affect testosterone levels including hereditary, environmental, psychosocial and socioeconomic factors. The Andropause is probably not related solely to declines in testosterone levels. Other hormones such as growth hormone and DHEA (a precursor of testosterone) are also decreased with aging.

Denial

If there is indeed a male menopause or Andropause, why is it that physicians do not promote treatment for the Andropause, as they enthusiastically do for the menopause? After all, older men also suffer from osteoporosis just like older women. Men rarely go on calcium or bone supplements called biphosphonates, let alone hormonal replacement. Research has shown that women may even delay the onset of dementia with estrogen replacement. Can the same be achieved for men? I am personally interested in pursuing the truths in this area.

Part of the reason that the Andropause is not widely recognized by doctors is that they were never taught its existence. There is no curriculum in medical school or residency to address this deficiency. The scientific literature in this area is also lacking. A quick check with Pub Med (the most reputable internet medical literature search engine developed by the NIH) reveals very little peer-reviewed research in this area. The research of Dr. Vermuelen from Belgium and my own seem to be the few scientific evaluations of the Andropause. The reason for little research in this area is the tragic lack of funding into the Andropause. I am personally unaware of any grants currently being directed towards research of the Andropause. This contrasts greatly with what is available in terms of funding for the menopause. Part of my reason of writing this book is to inform readers like yourself of this great discrepancy. The lack of knowledge amongst doctors themselves is contributing to the lack of recognition of this entity. As a result, the male patient suffers quietly.

Men themselves may fail to recognize that the Andropause is indeed a phenomenon. Part of the reason is because of the psyche of males. Men are, by and large, less likely to report symptoms than women. This has been substantiated in many studies. They believe they should be "macho" and the thought of losing their maleness scares them to death. There is great denial of the Andropause among some men. This seems to be related to educational levels and exposure to clinical information. Carefully treated, men can benefit from an improved quality of life in their Andropause years and beyond.

Andropause misunderstood

Some physicians adamantly deny the existence of the Andropause. My stand on this is that---- sorry, it DOES exist! How do I know? My patients strongly testify to it. I published a paper in the Archives of Andrology in 1999. About 30% of the 300 male patients that were interviewed said that they had experience the Andropause at some point in their lives. Perhaps, the group of patients who were interviewed had sampling bias, as they were all war veterans, most of whom had smoked and consumed alcohol heavily. I personally believe that in general, about a third to half of all men suffer from symptoms related to Andropause at some point in their lives. We know from studies that approximately 30% of men above 65 are hypogonadic or have low testosterone levels.

Andropause has been misunderstood by all, both by physicians as well as patients themselves. Many physicians fail to recognize this syndrome, and often misdiagnose it for something else. Of course the other extreme of over-diagnosing it is also incorrect, as when one attributes the complications of diabetic autonomic neuropathy to the Andropause. In addition, as previously stated, missing infectious disease like TB or malaria is totally unfair to the patient.

Opportunists also take advantage of the helpless andropausal man. Many herbal medications have been marketed to help treat erectile dysfunction but which have no scientific validity. There are shameless quacks are out there offering to treat and manage the Andropause, but who have no legitimacy. Tragically, the Andropause is badly misunderstood and there should be a crusade for a deeper and clearer understanding for all.

Chapter 2:
Aging Men and the Testosterone Story

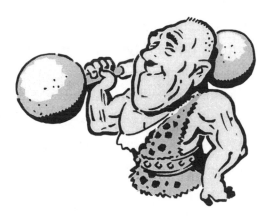

The theories of aging

Aging is inevitable because death is inevitable. In a sense we should consider ourselves fortunate, as man has never lived so long before. Life span has increased because of advances in medicine. Primarily, it has been good public health programs such as community vaccinations, hygienic water and better sanitation that have prolonged the human lifespan. However, with increasing lifespan also comes a prolonged period of decreased functionality. The organs in our body are forced to work those extra days, which was not the case for man living in the last century. For instance the average life span for men in Victorian England was about 45 years. Today, men live well into their seventies, eighties and even nineties.

The organs like the heart, brain, musculature and blood vessels take their toil with aging. The heart for instance becomes weaker and is not capable of pumping out as much blood as before. Fluid begins to accumulate in the legs and even in the lungs, resulting in heart failure. The brain cells or neurons die and become less capable of cognitive processes. Muscles atrophy and become weak, leading to difficulty walking and even falls. As bone becomes weaker with age, falls often lead to fractures. Blood vessels become less elastic with age and with the build up of cholesterol leads to raised blood pressures and events such as heart attacks and strokes.

There are many theories as to why we age. Arguably, the most favored theory is the gene regulation theory. It is believed that aging results because genes express themselves differently, especially after reproductive maturity. Andropause and menopause mark the end of a reproductive life, and thereafter, the genes we have express themselves differently. Genes control the production of proteins, and it is believed that this regulation is altered with aging. This occurs because genes that previously instructed protein to develop in a certain way stop doing so, and start producing a bad or ineffective protein. As you know, protein is essential for development of major parts of the body, including nerve cells, blood vessels and skin. As we age, our cells cannot repair themselves so effectively and this causes many of the problems of aging including vascular diseases and degeneration of nerves. Testosterone and estrogens along with some other hormones can reverse some of these changes in the post-andropausal or post-menopausal years.

It has been observed that longevity is related to the repair of DNA. Species that can repair DNA tend to live longer. For instance, elephants are remarkable in the sense that they can repair broken DNA easily, while this is not the case for flies. However, this theory is not highly favored, as there is no evidence in humans of a failure in the DNA repair system. As an alternative, the molecular theory of aging has been hypothesized which implicates the occurrence of translation errors. Translation is a step in the making of protein, and errors would result in defective muscles, blood vessels and nervous tissues. An immunology theory of aging also exists whereby it is believed that the immune system shuts down with aging. This is interesting, as testosterone has been shown in experiments to modulate the immune system. This may explain why testosterone could potentially be a hormone for the "fountain of youth".

Finally, one very popular theory that exists is the "free radical theory". It is believed that super oxide radicals can react with DNA, RNA, proteins and lipids. This leads to cellular damage and thus aging. This theory is very popular, as antioxidants such as Vitamin C and E have been shown in experiments to protect cells from oxidative damage. Many of you reading this book may already be taking both Vitamins C and E, and the reason why you are doing so is to prevent aging because of the "free radical theory".

What are hormones and what do they do?

I have just bought a can of fuel additive for my car. What a great analogy! I guess you can consider this additive as a form of hormonal supplement for the car. Our body produces hormones and these help to keep our bodily engine in optimal performance. Underproduction of most hormones slows us down, but excesses could be even more problematic. An example is the condition thyrotoxicosis or hyperthyroidism, whereby there is an excess of the hormone thyroxine. Thyroxine is produced by the thyroid glands, which are situated in the neck region. The thyroid controls the metabolic function of the body. When one is low on thyroid, this condition is called hypothyroidism. A hypothyroid patient becomes sluggish, puts on weight, is constipated and cold intolerant. Excess of thyroid hormone is called hyperthyroidism. In this condition when the patient becomes "hyper-metabolic". The patient has excessive energy, sweats profusely, loses weight and may even become neurotic. I guess that may be what happens when you put 90% fuel additive in your tank and only 10% regular gasoline!

There are other hormones in the body. They all work in union, and can be considered as members of an orchestra. The players are the different hormones and an orchestra conductor controls them. The hypothalamus regulates the pituitary gland, which in turn regulates several organs through hormones. Going back to the thyroid example, thyrothrophin-releasing hormone (TRH) is produced in the brain by the hypothalamus, and acts on the anterior part of the pituitary gland. The pituitary then produces thyroid stimulating hormone (TSH) which in turn stimulates the thyroid gland. Thyroxine (T4) converts to triiodothyroxine (T3) and act on various organs including the brain, nervous system, bowels, heart and thus explains the symptoms of over or underproduction as discussed above. Aging is associated with a decline in the ability to produce T3 from T4.

Various hormones control the sexual function of man. The hypothalamus secretes gonadotrophin-releasing hormone (GRH), which stimulates the pituitary gland. The pituitary gland responds by releasing follicular stimulating (FSH) and Luteinizing hormone (LH). FSH and LH then act on the target organs, in this case the testes, which then produces testosterone. The adrenal glands situated just above the kidneys also produce a small amount of testosterone. So, as you can imagine, in castrated males, the testosterone level fall dramatically. It is interesting that the State of California legislates castration as a form of punishment for sex offenders. On the flip side, doctors sometimes recommend castration as a means of treatment for advanced prostate cancer.

There are many other hormones that help keep us in balance. Other hormones such as insulin, growth hormone and melatonin manage the so-called homeostatic balance. Hormones such as antidiuretic hormone and aldosterone manage salt and water balance. The declines of some of these hormones occur during the aging process.

Replacement of these hormones can restore vitality. In fact, if properly supervised, these hormones can be considered as yet more "fountains of youth". However, they must be given under strict supervision and only when levels are inadequate. These hormones are powerful agents and if abused, can lead to multiple problems. Consider the disaster that will happen to your engine in the long run if you have 90% additive and only 10% gasoline in the fuel tank.

Lessons that may be learned from castration

The effects of castration have been known for a long time. Castration, the removal of the testes, essentially reduces most of the available source of testosterone. As early as in fourth century B.C., Aristotle, the great philosopher and scientist understood the physiological consequences of male castration. He recorded that "Following castration, some animals change their form and character. Men, if you mutilate them in boyhood, the later-growing hair never comes, and the voice never changes but remains high pitched. If they were mutilated in early manhood, the later growth of hair denies them except hair on the groin, and that diminishes but does not depart entirely. The congenital growth of hair never falls out, for a eunuch never goes bald. In the case of all castrated or mutilated male quadrupeds, the voice changes to a feminine voice. All animals, if operated on when they are young, become bigger and better looking than their unmutilated fellows."

A Christian sect called the Skopsy practiced castration as a path to holiness. This sect originated in Russia and spread to countries like Romania. The eunuchs of the China during the Qing dynasty were also castrated as a prerequisite to work in the imperial courts.

Castration was done in those days in a manner considered most barbaric by today's standards. The method performed on the eunuchs of China is described. Two assistants held the spread legs of the subject, while a third assistant secured the arms. The surgeon stood between the legs with a curved knife, grasped the scrotum and penis with his left hand and removed them with a curved knife upon consent either by the subject or the parent of the subject standing close by. A plug of pewter was introduced into the urethra (where the urine comes out) to prevent stricture (tightening) of the urethra. The wound was washed three times with a solution of boiled pepper and covered with a piece of soft, moist paper. With the support of two assistants, the subject is made to walk around the room for 2 hours. For the following 3 days, the subject is not allowed to drink liquids or urinate. On the fourth day, the dressing and plug were then removed. Healing took about 100 days. Many eunuchs suffered complications of urinary tract infections, incontinence and in some cases retention.

Much has been learnt from these groups of unfortunate men, as medical doctors and other scholars have observed the effects of testosterone deprivation. It is interesting that many of these events are also manifested in the post-andropausal stage in men, during which a natural "castration" occurs. In medical studies, several outcomes following castration in males have been documented:

1. There is enlargement of the pituitary gland. As explained earlier, the pituitary is the conductor of the hormonal orchestra.

2. There are skeletal changes. The younger castrated male grows very tall because there is failure of fusion of the epiphyses or the growth plates of his bones, the fusion process being dependent on testosterone. When they grew older, these castrated men experienced bone loss in the form of kyphosis (bending of the spine).

3. There is swelling of the breast or gynaecomastia. Following castration, profoundly low testosterone levels cause extra-glandular aromatization of adrenal androgens. As a result, increased estrogen is formed, and this is sufficient to cause breast enlargement. However not all castrated men were observed to have gynaecomastia.

4. There is disappearance of the prostate. Low testosterone levels lead to shrinking and ultimately missing prostates. Prostate cancer is believed in some circles to be related to high levels of testosterone. However, whether testosterone replacement directly cause prostate cancer is unclear at this point in time.

Hopefully, we will never again repeat the inhumane observational studies of castration. Nonetheless, the findings of those early physicians and scholars of the effects of castration have allowed us to deepen our understanding of the natural process of the Andropause. I believe that the Andropause is a form of natural castration that occurs with time, slowly but surely, in men.

Dr. Brown Sequard and his testosterone experiment

Every medical student is familiar with Dr. Brown Sequard, the eminent neurologist in the nineteenth century who first described the Brown Sequard Syndrome, a neurological condition sustained after injury to the spinal cord. The great bedside skills of observation that Dr. Brown Sequard had can be considered to surpass even the diagnostic accuracy of today's MRI scanners. His remarkable studies and analyses still continue to intrigue physicians of today. Towards the end of his life, Dr. Brown Sequard did an experiment on himself. He was 72 years old then, and quite frail. He decided to inject himself with a liquid that contained testosterone, and wrote the results of his experiment in the July 20, 1889 issue of the Lancet. The Lancet remains one of the most prestigious medical journals and stand in the company of journals such as the British Medical Journal, Journal American Medical Association and the New England Journal of Medicine. To fully appreciate his work and the potential role of testosterone, let me quote some of his excerpts written more than one hundred years ago.

"I have made use, in subcutaneous injections, of a liquid containing a small quantity of water mixed with the following three parts: first, blood of the testicular veins; secondly, semen; and thirdly, juice extracted from a testicle, crushed immediately after it has been taken from a dog or a guinea pig. The experiments, so far, do not allow of a positive conclusion as regards the relative power of the liquid obtained from a dog and that drawn from guinea pigs. All I can assert is that the two kinds of animals have given a liquid endowed with great power. I have hitherto made ten subcutaneous injections of a liquid – two in my left arm, all others in my lower limbs...

I am seventy-two years old. My general strength, which has been considerable, has notably and gradually diminished during the last ten to twelve years. The day after the first subcutaneous injection, and more after two succeeding ones, a radical change took place in me, and I had ample reason to say and write that I had regained the strength I possessed a good many years ago. After the second injection I found that I had fully regained my old powers, and returned to my previous habits in that respect. My limbs tested with a dynamometer, for a week before my trial and during the month following my first injection, showed a decided gain of strength. The average length of the jet of urine during the ten days that preceded the first injection was inferior by at least one quarter of what it came to be during the twenty following days. It is therefore quite evident that the power of the spinal cord over the bladder was considerably increased. After the first days of my experiments I have had a greater improvement with regard to the expulsion of fecal matters than in any other function.

With regard to the facility of intellectual labor, which had diminished within the last few years, a return to my previous ordinary condition became manifest during and after the first two or three days of my experiments...
I ceased making use of them for the purposes of ascertaining how long their good effects last. I have witnessed a complete return to the state of weaknesses, which existed before the first injection. My first communication to the Paris Biological Society was made with the wish that other medical men advanced in life would make on themselves experiments similar to mine..."

Those were rather haunting words of the great Dr. Brown Sequard. Although a hundred years have passed, not much more research has been done to reconfirm those preliminary findings, even though we have better preparations of testosterone, better biotechnology and obviously better scientific methods

Testosterone and moods

Mood disorders include conditions such as anxiety, depression, neurosis and some psychosis. It has been known for a long time that mood disorders can result from changes in the endocrine systems. Physicians commonly prescribe steroids for medical conditions, including emphysema, asthma, arthritis and immunological disorders. Patients treated with steroids may manifest the side effect of depression at one extreme, or euphoria at the other extreme.

Although there is little information on the behavioral effects of testosterone in humans, depression has been correlated with low levels of testosterone. A researcher in Alaska noted that as the days got shorter in winter, depression became more common. Interestingly, he also noted that as days got shorter, testosterone levels seemed to fall as well. He found a correlation of moods with testosterone levels and concluded that testosterone was essential to maintain happy moods. Cowley in an article in Newsweek (1996) reported that he himself felt much better after testosterone supplementation.

Unfortunately, the correlation of moods with depression is not very clear. Studies in young hypogonadic men treated with testosterone have shown improvement in mood, but studies in elderly men are sadly lacking. In females, we note that excess testosterones in women causes a condition called hirsutism, whereby there is excess hair growth in the male distribution, such as the upper lip & chin, and even chest. There is often a higher rate depression. Perhaps, testosterone does well for men in elevating their moods but does the reverse for women. My belief is that depression in older men could result from the loss of functionality, such as not being able to drive, walk or have sex. Testosterone may reverse some of the depression by improving functionality in the first instance. When one is able to walk again and regain one's sexuality, often the depression quickly goes too. In other words, testosterone may work indirectly to improve depression.

Testosterone and cognition

I strongly believe that testosterone is involved in the processing of memory. Along with other hormones, it is responsible for modulating and regulating the way the brain works through interacting with neurochemicals. Much can be learned from studies in animals. In several experiments, rats that were castrated lost their ability to navigate around mazes. These are crude experiments but may be the basis for more advanced work in this area. I have treated demented hypogonadic men with testosterone and have demonstrated improvements in their cognitive function. In particular the ability to perceive form, symmetry and space were improved. Scientifically, we call this portion of brain function the visual-spatial skills. Visual-spatial skills allow us to drive to work and play every day. We often take it for granted. When we loose the ability of visual- spatial cognition, we loose the dimension of space and time. We get lost trying to get from one place to another. We even cannot figure out the speedometer and end up in trouble. In a way, when we loose our testosterone, we become like the castrated mice in the maze- running and perspiring but not getting any where. Testosterone replacement holds a tremendous potential for unlocking the modulation of cognitive function, and in the future if funding for larger clinical trials are supported, this may prove to be a useful treatment for cognitive loss.

Testosterone and libido

How libido relates to testosterone levels is unclear. Anecdotally, I have seen and heard some of my patients report improvement in their libido following treatment with testosterone. There are also many reports of individuals who wrote on their improved libido following testosterone or DHEA treatments. One such example was Cowley who wrote in a Newsweek article (1996) of improved libido following treatment with androgens. A long-term prospective study of physiological and behavioral effects of hormone replacement in hypogonadic men suggest that sexual function is related to androgen status.

The largest database on male aging was conducted in New England and is currently on going. The data from the Massachusetts Aging Study (MMAS) essentially found no correlation between impotence and testosterone levels. However, they did find decreased levels of testosterone with aging. Sexual function correlated with the free or unbound portion of testosterone, and not with total testosterone levels.

To sum it up, it is controversial at this point to link testosterone levels with libido. However, testosterone may improve libido in some cases but not all. Libido is dependent on many factors and not to testosterone alone. It could be related to other neuro- chemicals such as epinephrine, serotonin and endorphin. Endorphins are naturally occurring opiates produce by the body. It helps the body preserve against pain and may also be responsible for libido.

Mr. D

I wish to describe a patient to illustrate a point about libido. Mr. D was a patient of mine diagnosed to have Alzheimer's dementia. He was able to mumble some words and would pace up and down all the time with seemingly endless energy. He was forgetful, but remained much to himself and was considered to be a nice person.

As he had low testosterone levels, he entered a clinical trial on the efficacy of testosterone in improving his cognitive functions. Two weeks following his first testosterone injection, his cognitive functions were measurably better. He was able to reproduce the clock face (a test for spatial-spatial ability) better than he could before. However, we got a side effect of testosterone that we never quite anticipated. His libido improved so tremendously that he became hypersexual! He even approached several nurses with inappropriate requests. So in a sense, I can say testosterone does improve libido in *some* individuals!

Testosterone and osteoporosis

Peak bone mass in men is achieved at age 25 to 29 years and declines gradually after that. It is reported in cross sectional studies that typically, vertebral bone loss in healthy men is 1.2% per year. Elderly men have hip fracture rates and vertebral fracture rates that are at least half those of women. Then, as more and more testosterone is lost, especially in the very elderly, fractures become even more common in these hypogonadic men. Hence, after 80 years of age, fracture rates in men equal that of women.

However, the subject of osteoporosis in men receives little attention in contrast to osteoporosis in women. As testosterone is lost gradually, men are somewhat less vulnerable than women, who suddenly loose most of their estrogens at the time of menopause. Interestingly, several large epidemiological studies have found that in aging men, bone mineral density correlates better with serum estrogen (the female hormone) than testosterone. The reason may be that testosterone is aromatized to estradiol (which is an estrogen) as one ages. Despite this fact, testosterone replacement as a treatment of osteoporosis in men should still be considered, as eventually, testosterone in the body gets converted to estrogens. If you recall, I started the book by describing a patient of mine that regained bone strength following testosterone replacement. He had broken his arm merely from being held up by the nursing aides - unbelievable but true!

Testosterone and blood cell production

Blood is produced in areas like the kidneys, spleen and the bone marrow. In certain disease states like kidney failure, there is a failure to produce red blood cells, which is one of the components of blood.

Testosterone modulates the production of blood. One of the side effects of testosterone is excess red blood cells or polycythemia. Testosterone stimulates the kidneys to produce erythropoietin, the hormone that stimulates red blood cell production. In advanced kidney failure erythropoietin production is reduced, and hence, artificial erythropoietin (Epogen) is sometimes given to kidney failure patients in an attempt to stimulate red cell production. At this time, testosterone does not have FDA approval for treatment of anemia related to kidney failure, but I wish to use the following case to illustrate this beneficial effect of testosterone.

Mr. R

Mr. R was seeing me for multiple illnesses. He had high blood pressure and diabetes that had affected his kidneys. In fact his kidneys failed to a point where he needed dialysis. I had questioned his sexual function after undergoing surgical castration for advanced cancer of the prostate. He also had lost weight and was depressed. After starting him on testosterone, some of his weight returned in the form of muscle. Also, he began to smile a bit more and

45

became more open about his illness. I had also improved his blood count with the testosterone treatment. Initially, this was not planned. Testosterone was meant for another reason, but his blood system benefited. Paradoxically, a side effect of the medication, increasing the red cells, proved to be therapeutic for Mr. R's anemia, which was due to his kidneys failing.

Testosterone and the heart

This is a very controversial area. Some of my colleagues working in this area have found no untoward effects of testosterone on the heart. In a study of 11 men by Dr. K.C. Tan (no relation of mine) receiving testosterone injections, no significant changes in plasma cholesterol was found. However, testosterone has been shown in other studies to affect the fat metabolism in the body. The good cholesterol (HDL) has been shown to decrease in animals receiving testosterone, while the bad cholesterol (LDL) increased. The significance of these animal studies is not clear. Women have lower cardiovascular illnesses before the menopause, and estrogens seem to be protective in the pre- menopausal stages. Some studies have shown that testosterone narrows arteries in the heart, but conversely, other studies have demonstrated that testosterone opens the coronary arteries. Thus whether testosterone protects or harms the heart in men is unclear.

Testosterone and autoimmune disorders

Autoimmune disorders are illnesses that result because your body produces antibodies that attack the cells of your own body. Examples include rheumatoid arthritis, autoimmune thyroiditis and systemic lupus erythematosus (SLE). Testosterone may have a role in autoimmune disorders, because most of the effects of androgens on the immune system are suppressive. Studies on rats show protective effects of testosterone against experimental autoimmune thyroiditis and SLE. Interestingly, rheumatoid arthritis and SLE are more common in women than men. Perhaps, androgens protect men from these diseases. It has been suggested that men who develop SLE may have a relative shortage of testosterone. Male patients with rheumatoid disease have benefited from treatment with testosterone. Likewise, testosterone has been shown to improve quality of life by slowing the disease in patients with AIDS, as it is known that testosterone builds up muscle in the wasting syndrome of AIDS.

Testosterone and muscle

The effect of testosterone on muscle can be harnessed for rehabilitating disused muscles that come with aging. One of the first successful experiments was carried out by a physician, Dr. Brown Sequard, on himself, as described earlier. In recent years, Emory University conducted a placebo controlled double blind randomized trial and measured the effects of testosterone on muscle and functional activities of daily living. Muscle strength improved in the treated group but not in the group that was given placebo. The treated group also improved functionally. The trial was short-term but testosterone proved to be safe and effective. I have personally witnessed many patients that have become stronger and improved their mobility.

Mr. LC

Mr. LC was 75 years old, married and crippled with arthritis. He mobilized with a walker. He came to see me essentially for control of his diabetes and high blood pressure. On routine questioning, I asked if he had symptoms pertaining to the Andropause. He gave a 5-year history of night sweats, 10 years of erectile dysfunction and some recent memory loss. I thought he fit into the classical picture of the Andropause. This was confirmed on blood testing:

> Total testosterone 190ng/dL (normal 241-827)
> Free testosterone 24.4ng/dL (normal 9-25)
> FSH 9.6 mIU/mL (normal 1-8.0)
> LH 3.8 mIU/mL (normal 2.0- 12.0)

As explained in an earlier chapter, low testosterone levels with an elevated FSH clinch the diagnosis. He was started on intramuscular testosterone 200mg, and after 2 weeks came back to see me.

I was astonished. Here was a different man - he was walking straight and without his walker! He was smiling and seemed happy. I asked him how he was. He replied, " You have made me a new man. See - I am walking without my walker, and I believe my memory is better. I even had an erection the other night. I am so pleased!"

Testosterone and the prostate

This is another area of controversy, similar to the issue of whether breast cancer can result from estrogen replacement. To date, this is unclear and we have experts giving contradicting opinions. As for testosterone, there are several studies that suggest that testosterone is safe in the short-term and that it does not cause cancer of the prostate. Admittedly, there have been individual case reports of prostate cancer in patients following treatment with testosterone. What is unknown in those case reports was whether there was already subclinical prostate cancer even before treatment with testosterone. In any case, the scientific literature does suggest that topical testosterone is less likely to increase PSA levels (a prostate cancer screening test) as compared to injectable testosterone. In other words, it may be safer to use topical testosterone.

Mr. C

Mr. C was another nursing home patient of mine. He had multiple problems, including advanced cancer of the prostate that was in remission following a surgical castration. One of the treatments for advanced metastatic cancer of the prostate is the removal of the testes by surgery. This may seem a cruel operation but it is sometimes necessary in order to contain a devastating disease. You may recall that the testes are the main sites of production of testosterone. Without testosterone, his bones became very brittle, his memory failed and he became very weak. Testosterone replacement was carefully discussed with him after explaining fully the risks involved, including possible recurrence of his prostate cancer. After 2 months of therapy, Mr. C started having his erections again, and he was notably stronger and able to ambulate again. Unfortunately, Mr. C did pass away, not from his prostate cancer but of a raging pneumonia, which was unrelated to both the testosterone treatment and his prostate cancer. I brought him up as a case for discussion, as men rarely get testosterone replacement after surgical castration, for fear of recurrence of prostate cancer. Paradoxically, after removal of the uterus and ovaries as in a total hysterectomy and oophorectomy, it is standard practice to replace estrogens without thinking twice. Physicians don't fear that estrogens could lead to increase risk of beast cancers. Why shouldn't testosterone replacement be considered more often for men? Perhaps there are some sexist views existing in our times.

In my personal experience, I have yet to see any case of prostate cancer induced by testosterone replacement. However, I always carefully screen the patient to make sure that he does not have prostate cancer before instituting treatments with testosterone, including performing a digital examination and checking for a normal PSA level.

A concept often practiced in medicine is "cost versus benefit" analysis. Is the cost of treatment likely to outweigh the benefit reaped by the patient? The cost could be a direct cost, such as the price of the medication. The cost could also be indirect, such as any harm or discomfort caused to the patient. Testosterone is cheap, costing a few dollars a shot. The benefits are tremendous, and hidden behind all this is a remote possibility of prostate cancer. I often discuss this concept with my patients before starting treatments, as informed consent is always important in good medical practice.

Chapter 3:
My Research
on the Andropause

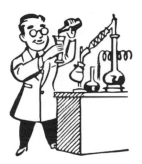

The state of affairs on the Andropause

Since the age of 3 when I got trapped in my mum's dryer –
at least it was not on, I always had an enquiring mind, and
have been involved in medical research for about 15 years. I
had focused previously on depression in older patients- a
very gloomy area of research indeed. After a lot of hard
work, some of my articles were published in well-to-do
international journals including the British Journal of Clinical
Pharmacology, the Journal of the American Geriatrics Society
(JAGS), the British Medical Journal (BMJ) and the Journal
American Medical Association (JAMA). Modesty apart, I have
also written reviews for Postgraduate Medicine, Clinical
Geriatrics and several other medical journals.

When I first got interested in the Andropause a few years
ago, I embarked on a real, as well as a virtual, tour of the

medical libraries. You probably guessed what I found - not much at all! There were two main frustrations. Firstly, although there was a ton of research material on the Menopause, there was minimal on the Andropause. All I could find were review articles, as opposed to research articles, on this topic. Paradoxically I learned more from non-medical magazines like Esquire, Men's Health and Newsweek, than traditional medical sources. Secondly, there was even some confusion with the terminology of the male menopause. Some have called it Andropause, Viropause and even the Male Menopause. A recent article in the Journal of Urology aptly called this the ADAM - Androgen Decline in Aging Men. Clearly, there has to a consensus before we go any further.

Through my research I discovered some very salient points. Testosterone levels begin to decline at the age of 50, with the lowest levels in men above 70 years. The rate of decline in serum testosterone is gradual and is approximately 100ng/dl/decade. As mentioned in an earlier chapter, there is a compensatory rise in FSH and LH hormones in some men, just like that in the menopausal women. Estrogen levels seem to drop more dramatically at the time of Menopause than the corresponding fall of testosterone at the Andropause. Hence the rise in FSH and LH for females is more acute.

Environmental factors have been known to affect how the body function. Environmental factors, if modified, can result in better health status. I am referring to tobacco, alcohol and certain toxins in our environment. I came across some literature that linked an earlier onset of the Menopause to smoking. I hypothesized that the same effects of smoking on the onset of Andropause. This is possible because nicotine has been demonstrated to adversely affect gonadal tissue and hence, sexual function.

How the study was conducted

My study was conducted on men attending clinics in a medical center for various problems. I conducted a study that was, in epidemiological terms, a "non-experimental, cross-sectional study". This was because no drugs or intervention were used in this study, and we obtained data by conducting an interview with each subject. Altogether 22 questions were asked by a single interviewer to avoid inter-rater non-reliability. In other words, having the same interviewer improved accuracy. The ethics committee and the institutional review board, the watchdogs for research, approved the study. This was to ensure that our study was legitimate, and not harmful in any way to the health or privacy of our interviewees. Consent was also taken before we asked any questions, and the responses were all anonymous.

The questions I wanted answered

I wanted to find answers to several questions and collected the data for analysis using software with spreadsheet and statistical capabilities.

The data we collected fell into these domains:

1. Social demographic characteristics, which included information on the interviewee's ethnic origin.
2. The amount of cigarettes smoked and the amount of alcohol consumed.
3. Concomitant illnesses such as high blood pressure and diabetes were noted.
4. The interviewee was asked about his familiarity of the Andropause and whether he had experienced it.
5. If so, what symptoms did he think he had undergone during the Andropause.
6. The interviewee's knowledge and attitude of the Andropause were explored:
    a. Whether he thought he would be infertile during the Andropause
    b. Whether he thought he needed testosterone replacement during the Andropause
    c. Whether he thought there was a relationship of medications to impotency
    d. Questions pertaining to the utilization of health care services for problems related to the Andropause
    e. The issue of the legality of purchasing over-the-counter androgens like DHEA

Who were the patients?

I am always very thankful to my patients, as it is from them that I have learnt a tremendous amount. Without their help, much of this new knowledge would not be possible. The study would not be possible if not for their gracious participation.

Altogether 302 men were interviewed. Ninety eight percent of the men were above 40 years of age, with the largest group (71.8%) in the 60-80 years age range. This was the target group, because if Andropause were to occur, it would be in this age range. In my study, 87% of the interviewees were described as white, 6% Hispanics and 5% African Americans, 2% others including Asians and Native Americans.

What symptoms did the men associate with the Andropause?

The results of this study probably represents the first article published in a medical journal on the symptoms associated with the Andropause. Previously, most information on symptoms was based on anecdotal reports of men published in non-medical journals. The chart below shows the frequency of the symptoms of the Andropause, as reported by the study subjects.

In this study, impotence or erectile dysfunction was the most common symptom associated with Andropause.

Erectile dysfunction is the medical term for "failure to have a penile erection". Altogether 46% of the 302 men reported this symptom to be associated with the Andropause. It is interesting to note that not all men associated erectile dysfunction with the Andropause. Conversely in women, cessation of the menses is seen in ALL women who undergo Menopause.

The second most common symptom was weakness. Forty one percent of the 302 patients interviewed said this was a symptom associated with the Andropause. There could be many reasons for the weakness. It could be due to the real loss of muscle mass, as loss of testosterone has been demonstrated in studies to result in muscle weakness. Indeed, in a study at Emory University, muscle strength was regained after testosterone replacement. Another possible reason for some patients to report muscle weakness is that bone loss happens in the Andropause, as a result of declines in testosterone levels. Weaker bones subsequently cause muscle atrophy. I have demonstrated in studies that bone strength can be regained with testosterone replacement.

The third most common symptom was memory loss. It is not uncommon for patients who undergo the Andropause to report misplacing a key or forgotten important details. Often the memory loss is so minor it does not affect everyday functioning. This memory loss has sometimes been referred to as "age related memory loss" and is not quite the degree of Alzheimer's dementia. Memory loss in the andropausal years has been a research interest of mine. I have replaced testosterone in hypogonadic men who have dementia and have demonstrated improvements in their visual-spatial cognitive functions. The study results have been presented at several scientific meetings. Another researcher in Oregon has found similar results on improving cognitive functions with testosterone in normal older men.

Intimacy problems were reported by 11% of the men in this study. Intimacy problems relate to issues such as wanting to be closer to family members, for example one's children. It seems as if many men at this point begin to feel more "maternal" and this may be because of the relative loss of testosterone. During this time, some men also report spouse-related problems. Men at this time are reaching out for help in their relationships. They usually are quiet about it, but many need help desperately.

Only only a minority of men reported hot flashes, in contrast to the menopausal female - at the time of menopause, 9 out of 10 women report hot flashes. I believe the difference lies in the fact that the loss of testosterone is more gradual in men, whereas in women, estrogen loss occurs much more suddenly. Hence the autonomic nervous system is put into disarray all of a sudden for women, whereas in men, there is much more time to compensate. Sometimes, hot flashes are not noticed because men commonly describe a night sweats rather than hot flashes.

In my study, the age most commonly reported for the Andropause to occur was between *51 to 60 years*, as claimed by 38% of the study subjects. The next age group most likely to be associated with the Andropause was between *60 to 70 years*, as experienced by 26% of subjects.

Smaller groups reported that it occurred as young as between 40 to 50, or as late as in the eighties. About one in ten (11%) said that they were unsure if Andropause ever occurred. I suspect this 11% includes some men that had not undergone the Andropause yet.

What makes it more likely for some men to have the Andropause?

The 6 million dollar question has always been why do some men experience the Andropause, while others do not? Why are some men protected and why is it that in some men, the testosterone levels fall much more rapidly than in others? All women undergo the menopause at a point in their lives, but they do report different symptoms. Some just get very mild hot flashes and irritability, but others are so troubled that they fall into bleak depression.

So far, there have been no large epidemiological studies to determine the true rate of the Andropause. My small database of 302 men does give us some clues. Only 30% of the 302 men reported that they had awareness of the Andropause, and had personally experienced it at some point in their lives. Seventy percent said that they had not even come across the word "Andropause". This could mean several things. It could be that within this group of 70%, some had already experienced the Andropause without knowing it, while others in this group had not experienced it yet. Research has shown that men are less likely to present with symptoms of disease as compared to women, and tend to be more insular in this respect. My study suggests that 1 in 3 men undergo Andropause at some point in their lives, but my gut feeling tells me that the true prevalence reaches 1 in 2. This correlates with the results of studies on the prevalence of hypogonadism (low testosterone) in older men. Most studies suggest a prevalence rate of hypogonadism in older men (above 65) to be 30-50%. That may be an alarming statistic especially with the world population aging so rapidly!

My suspicion of smoking and the Andropause

In recent years, much has been exposed of the harmful effects of smoking. It is known to contribute towards heart disease, lung disease and strokes. Some cancers are attributed to the nicotine found in cigarettes. The scientific literature reveals that women who smoke tend to have an earlier onset of menopause. In a study on Czech women, females that smoked more than 5 cigarettes a day had an average age of menopause at 49.5 years, the norm being 51 years. That study also found that 1.5 years of fertile life is lost to smoking. Other studies performed in the United States and Mexico also revealed similar results.

In my study the average age that Andropause occurred was 55 years. However, in those who smoked more than 10 cigarettes a day, the average age of presentation was 50 years. How smoking affects the onset of Andropause is unclear, and obviously more research is needed in this direction. It has been suggested that smoking can have a negative effect on gonadotrophin releasing hormone (GnRH) pulse generator, which is secreted from the hypothalamus and acts on the pituitary gland to produce LH and FSH. These in turn act on the gonads to produce testosterone. Lowered testosterone levels have been associated with the onset of andropausal symptoms. In short, smoking may inhibit the release of GnRH, which ultimately lowers the testosterone levels.

Impotence during the Andropause and the need for testosterone replacement

It is interesting to note that almost half (48%) of the men we interviewed admitted to having problems with impotence. However, many patients believe that they maintain reproductive lives till the time of the Andropause.

In my survey, I asked the question: "Do you think your impotence may be related to low testosterone levels?" About half (51%) said they were not sure. This response probably reflects the present state of knowledge of the relationship between impotence and testosterone levels. The Massachusetts Aging Study found no correlation of impotence to testosterone levels. Many doctors treat impotence and erectile dysfunction with testosterone without even measuring levels of testosterone. With this thought in mind, I went on to ask patients another question - "If the doctor told you that your testosterone levels were normal, would you still want a testosterone shot?" The response surprised me. Again almost half (48%) said YES, implying that there is never too much of a good thing! In medical practice, we tend to replace electrolytes, hormones and so on only if they are low. This practice makes good sense – you replace calcium if it is low, and you replace thyroxine if the thyroid is non-functioning. This is analogous to filling your gas tank only if it is empty.

However, when it comes to testosterone, men have a different perception. They believe that excessive levels may increase sexual prowess! In fact, several anti-aging physicians also believe in this concept, although unfortunately this has never been scientifically verified and would be an interesting research question. Today, even women take testosterone, especially in the post-menopausal years to improve libido.

Utilization of health-care services for problems related to the Andropause

Women today have very well established preventive programs for the menopause. Typically, a woman will get breast exams, mammography, PAP smears and even estrogen replacement. Men do not have such programs, especially post-andropausal men. Patients may occasional see their doctors for erectile dysfunction, but usually that symptom is left to the last, after consulting for the more conventional symptoms such as blood pressure, cholesterol and pain.

I wanted to study the utilization of existing services related to the Andropause. Only 20% of subjects said that there were currently adequate services to provide for the care of andropausal men. Alarmingly, 80% said that not enough was being done, and 70% were in favor of "men's clinic" to address issues of the Andropause. There is an immense void out there, and more funding to support such programs is badly needed.

Consuming non-prescription drugs such as DHEA

At the time of writing, DHEA or Dihydoepiandrostenedione, is easily available over the counter. This should be considered a form of testosterone, because it is a precursor of testosterone. In other words, it becomes testosterone after breaking down in the body. It does have some of the potency of testosterone and with it, the potential side effects.

As this "super vitamin" is easily available over the counter without a prescription or a doctor's supervision, I wanted to explore what patients thought of it. I asked the question, "Is it legal for you to obtain hormones without a prescription over the counter?" Again, the results surprised me. Forty percent said it was all right, and implied that many were already doing so. Today, many hormones can be bought over the Internet without questions. Hormones like testosterone are powerful drugs, and the administration has to be carefully monitored. I will discuss the potential side effects of testosterone in a later chapter.

Abstracts of some of my scientific presentations for readers interested in the scientific medical literature

Abstract 1 - Pathological Fracture due to Testosterone deficiency in an Elderly Man

A 76-year-old man was transferred to our nursing home for rehabilitation after sustaining a fracture of the right humerus in the hospital. He did *not* have a fall, but broke his arm while being transferred to the toilet. The patient has no alcohol history, is not on steroids and never had gastric surgery or disturbances in calcium metabolism. On physical examination, he appeared cherubic, and pale looking. There was bruising over the entire right arm and was very tender over the mid humerus. The abdomen was protuberant, and bowel sounds were normal. An important finding was the *absence* of pubic and axillary hair. His testes were descended and small. The prostate was normal size and of a firm consistency.

Important laboratory & radiological findings include: 1) Hgb= 13 g/dl, MCV= 97.1 fl, WBC= 5.9 k/cumm 2) Urea= 29 mg/dl, Cr= 2 mg/dl, Alk PO4= 119 IU/L 3) Serum Ca= 9.3 mg/dl, Urinary Ca= 5.9 mg/dl, total in 24 hrs. = 132 mg/dl (100-300) 4) FSH= 0.5 mg/dl (<16), LH= 0 mg/dl (11.3- 56.4), *Testosterone=*

88 ng/dl (241- 827), TSH= 2.18 mcIU/L. Xray right arm showed a comminuted fracture and generalized osteopenia . Skeletal bone scans no evidence of lytic process thus suggesting no metastatic bone disease.

We concluded that his hypogonadic status was contributory to his pathological fracture, as he did not have any other secondary cause of osteoporosis. On direct questioning, the patient confessed to having problems with his libido and requested treatment for it. We started him on im testosterone 200mg q 2 weeks. Baseline measures included his MMSE= 24/30, GDS= 5/15, MADRS= 6/30, FIM= 98/126 and will be repeated after 2 months. Subjectively, he reported better health, and was stronger. He was also seen to be mobilizing more independently. However, he did *not* report improvement in his libido. Repeat X rays have confirmed healing of the fracture of the humerus.

This is an unusual case of a pathological fracture from secondary osteoporosis as a result of hypogonadism. A lesson learnt from this case is that a *complete physical examination* in every geriatric patient is essential. The hospital staff had unfortunately missed his hypogonadic status. Hypogonadism is a common occurrence in aging males and a prevalence of 20% in the elderly has been quoted. Chronic hypogonadism results in greater loss of bone mass and hence fractures. Male osteoporosis is an area not well researched and studied. Our case report may support the potential role of testosterone in the prevention of osteoporosis in elderly men. However, the risks/benefits ratio must always be considered.

Abstract 2 - Perceived memory loss in the Andropause

The Andropause seems to be less defined than the female Menopause. Our study on older patients describes how they perceive and understand this aging process.

We performed a non-interventional, cross-sectional study to determine what male patients report as symptoms of the andropause. In particular, we wanted to ascertain if memory loss was a predominant feature. Our hypothesis was that androgens, such as testosterone were responsible for visual-spatial and memory development. As such the aging process of andropause, which is associated with declines in testosterone levels would lead to memory loss. A standardized questionnaire of 22 questions was administered to 302 outpatients of a medical center. Information on patient demographics, understanding of the andropause, and concomitant risk factors were collected.

Of the 302 patients, 71% were above 60 years and whites predominated at 87%. Memory loss was reported in 36% of the patients who felt that they had experienced the andropause. It was the third most common symptom after erectile dysfunction (46%) and general weakness (41%). Twenty two percent of the 302 patients had a history of diabetes. Among those that reported to have undergone the andropause, diabetic patients were more likely to report memory loss (p= 0.03, OR= 1.9, CI= 1.1- 3.4). Sixty-four percent of patients reported the onset of andropause to be between 50-70 years (the median age being 50-60 years).

This study highlights the importance of testosterone in maintaining cognitive functions. It supports studies of testosterone replacement in men undergoing the andropause and who have concomitant dementia. This results parallel recent reports of the neuroprotective effects of estrogens in preventing dementia. We feel that diabetes is associated with memory loss in our study because of the additional insults to cognitive function of the brain secondary to ischemia.

Abstract 3 - Testosterone improves cognition in hypogonadic demented patients

---

Dementia is highly prevalent in nursing homes. The male aging process also brings about declines in hormonal function including testosterone levels. Studies suggest a link with estrogens and dementia. The role of testosterone is unclear. We hypothesized that testosterone replacement in elderly hypogonadic males may improve cognition, in particular visual-spatial.

The pilot study design was single blind and interventional in nature. Eighteen consecutive male patients with a diagnosis of dementia had their testosterone levels measured. Five patients of 18 (28%) were deemed biochemically hypogonadic (< 240 ng/dL). Initial MMSE ranged from 17 to 22. The Clock Drawing Test (CDT), being a good measure of visual-spatial abilities was used. Normal PSA levels were essential before treatments. The baselines were repeated at 3, 6 and 9 months of treatment with intramuscular testosterone 200 mg.

Results obtained were baseline mean testosterone=126.4 ng/dl, MMSE=19.4, CD=2.2, PSA=0.98. At 9 months of treatment, testosterone levels increased in the 5 patients from a mean of

68

126.4ng/dl to 341ng/dl (p= 0.11). PSA were also elevated from a mean of 0.98 to 1.37 (p= 0.07). MMSE improved from a mean of 19.4 to 23.2 (p= 0.02), CDT also improved from 2.2 to 3.2 (p= 0.03). Four of the 5 patients continued treatments beyond the 9 months; one was stopped because of hypersexual behavior.

This pilot study performed in male nursing home patients suggested that testosterone could indeed improve cognition, including visual-spatial skills in mild to moderate dementia. This could be due to the modulation of neurotransmitters by testosterone. The next step would be for a randomized, placebo-controlled double blind study to confirm these preliminary findings.

Abstract 4 - Attitudes of Older Males toward the Andropause

Male aging is associated with a series of clinical symptoms in the climacterium that may be analogous to the Menopause and is termed Andropause. The objective of our on-going study is to identify symptoms, delineate onset and evaluate male attitudes and familiarity with the Andropause. The study design was cross-sectional and was performed on patients attending clinics at the Medical Center.

Methodology involved an interview questionnaire instrument consisting of 22 characteristics. A single investigator, to attain consistency and optimize inter-rater reliability, interviewed 302 male patients. The study was conducted July through September 1997. Statistical analysis was performed using Chi-Square, Spearman correlation and logistic regression.

Over 70% of men surveyed were between the age of 60 and 80. Eighty seven percent were White, 6% Hispanic and 5% Black. Almost 70% were hearing of Andropause for the first time, and 85% had never visited a physician for problems relating to Andropause. Yet, almost 70% expressed interest in being educated about Andropause. Over 50% identified their onset of Andropause between the age of 50 and 70. However, *smoking* was independently associated with an earlier onset of Andropause before the age of 50 (logistic regression, p= 0.03). Symptoms of Andropause that were commonly reported included impotence (46%), weakness (41%) and memory loss (36%). However, *diabetes* was also independently associated with impotence (logistic regression, p= 0.01) and weakness (logistic regression, p= 0.002), as was *hypertension* with weakness (logistic regression, p=0.001). Surprisingly, 39.7% of the study population felt that they should be on testosterone replacement during the Andropause and 55.6% believed that testosterone should be taken even if they had normal levels. Fifty nine percent feel that it was illegal to buy androgens like DHEA over the counter without a prescription.

There is unfamiliarity with Andropause among survey participants, but a keen interest and perhaps a need for education about this entity. Smoking can be a risk factor for earlier onset of symptoms of Andropause.

Chapter 4:
Memory Loss in the Andropause

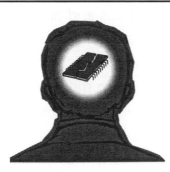

The mystery of Memory

Memory is a marvelous gift from God, and truly intriguing. Why is it that we can remember nursery rhymes or stories told to us in childhood? Why is it that driving seems automatic, and we can remember how to get to work and home every day without effort? On the other hand, why is it that we forget trivial details like what we had for breakfast 2 days ago? We take memory for granted and often appreciate it only when our own memories fail.

Memory is the process whereby information is retained in the mind. Somehow, our experiences are archived in the brain, and then recovered when we recall that information. Memory is also intimately associated with learning. It can be said that learning is the acquisition of new knowledge, whereas memory is the retention of learned knowledge.

These are two broad categories of memory, declarative memory and procedural memory. Declarative memory is the memory for facts and events, such as dates, historical facts and telephone numbers. Procedural memory is the memory for procedures and abilities, such as driving a car, playing football and brushing your teeth. In general, the order in which the different memory categories is lost is opposite to the order in which the memory categories were formed. Hence, declarative memory is generally lost earlier during the dementing process, and procedural memory later on. This is because procedural memory is usually developed before declarative memory, although sometimes both develop simultaneously. In the clinical setting, we measure procedural memory in terms of "Instrumental activities of Daily Living" (IADL), a scoring system which basically measures how well routine functions are conducted. Examples of IADLs are the ability to use the telephone, write checks, do the laundry and go grocery shopping. The IADLs decline when dementia sets in.

We sometimes remember things by forming ideas of shapes and sizes. We hear of people having a "photographic memory', as if the brain of that person actually takes a photograph of the event or the page in the book. Visual-spatial memory refers to the ability of the brain to remember dimensions and directions, and is often lost in early dementia. This results in the inability to perform certain

IADLs, and may cause a driver to get lost, or the inability to tell the time.

Let's say you meet someone new, and she tells you her name and phone number. After you shake hands and part company, how often is it that you say to yourself, "Shucks, now what was her name? And there's no way I will remember those numbers without having written them down!" You are engaging a form of memory that is temporary and limited in its capacity. It is stored for a very short time in the brain, in the order of a few seconds to minutes. This is called short-term memory. For short-term memory to become permanent, attention, repetition and associated ideas is required. To return to our example, let's say 2 weeks later while driving, you suddenly recall the name of the person you met, and you smile, "It was Lisa!" Subconsciously, the information had been stored in the long-term memory, which is more lasting and has a greater capacity. The process of storing new information in long-term memory is called consolidation. An elaboration of short-term memory is working memory. Working memory may have multiple sites in the brain where temporary storage occurs, rather than a single short-term memory system.

Why is it I cannot remember?

Memory is not situated in only one structure in the brain. It is important to learn about the different structures of the brain so as to understand how it works. Much information about where memory is stored was gleaned from studying animals who had parts of their brains removed, and from patients who underwent brain surgery to remove diseased parts because of accidents or cancer.

The temporal lobe is one region of the brain believed to store past memory, and in memory loss, there can be demonstrable loss of neuronal function in this area. Alzheimer's disease involves the "cortical" or superficial layers of the brain and, in later stages, can affect the temporal lobe.

The hippocampus assigns the locations where facts and events will be stored. It is also involved in the recognition of novelties and their spatial relations, such as the recognition of map directions. Declarative memory, such as for facts and events, seems to involve the hippocampus, the surrounding cortical structures, and its connections to other parts of the brain.

The amygdala is a "hub" for the brain. It communicates with the thalamus and other sensorial systems of the cortex through its extensive connections. Sound, smell, taste and touch become electrical signals in the amygdala that activate a circuit that is related to memory. Connections between the amygdala and the hypothalamus allow emotions to influence learning. The pre-frontal cortex also has an important role in the solving of problems and the planning of behavior.

Brain cells are called neurons and each neuron contributes to behavior and mental activity. Cellular alterations resulting from learning and memory are called plasticity. When we learn and remember, neurons interconnect with each other.

Many factors "regulate" how the brain remembers. Such factors include hormones, including estrogen and testosterone. Thus, in males with low testosterone levels, defects in memory can be present as the regulatory hormones are inadequate to help the neurons perform and interconnect as described above. Without hormones, the interconnections could be disrupted or lost. In my research, many men complained of memory problems in their post-andropausal years. It is unclear if testosterone plays a direct or indirect role in memory preservation. It may be that testosterone exerts its influence by converting first to estrogens. Memory can be improved in some hypogonadic men with testosterone. Later in this chapter, I will describe my findings of memory improvements in men who received testosterone replacement.

What is Dementia?

Many of us worry when we get older because we begin to feel that our memory is not as good as it used to be. Normal aging can be associated with slower thinking and poorer memory. Distinguishing age-related memory loss from that caused by a disease process such as dementia can be difficult, especially in the early stages.

For a patient to be diagnosed with dementia, there must be a decrease in the level of functioning, in addition to the impairment of the memory. This means that there is the inability to perform some activities of daily living such as handling personal finances, cooking, driving safely, and so on. These activities are usually performed effortlessly and subconsciously by normally functioning individuals. In the late stages of dementia, patients even lose their ability to care for themselves, and need assistance with feeding, bathing, using the bathroom and walking.

There are several theories as to how dementia develops. It may be genetically linked, caused by a slow virus, vascular insult, hormonal imbalance or merely a function of aging. In dementia, the nerve transmitters do not function adequately, leading to a failure of brain function. Several nerve transmitters are involved, and they include acetylcholine, norepinephrine , serotonin and a substance called GABA. In dementia, there is an excessive deposition of a substance called amyloid, leading to a failure of transmission of nerve impulses. Drugs developed today to combat dementia often increase nerve transmission by inhibiting the natural breakdown of the nerve transmitters.

The most common form of dementia is Senile Dementia of Alzheimer's Type, commonly known as Alzheimer's disease, which accounts for about 90% of cases. Approximately 5% of people older than 65, and 20% of people older than 85, have Alzheimer's disease. A smaller number of cases is due to multi-infarct dementia. In this form of dementia, the patient usually has a previous history of diabetes or hypertension, coupled with neurological findings or a fluctuating course of memory deficit. Rarer causes of dementia include Pick's Disease, Crutzfield Yacob's disease and brain tumors.

However, memory loss is not always Dementia!

Depression, hypothyroidism and certain medications are notorious for mimicking dementia, and this is referred to as pseudo-dementia, or false dementia. Consequently, when these underlying diseases are treated, the symptoms of "dementia" are correspondingly reversed. Sometimes, infections and electrolyte imbalance may also cause an elderly person to be confused and forgetful. The medical term for this condition is delirium, and again, the symptoms are reversed when the infection or electrolyte imbalance is treated.

How is Dementia diagnosed?

When one sees the physician to be evaluated for dementia, neuropsychological tests may be administered. This would involve the patient answering questions so that the physician can assess his memory, language skills, conceptualization process, visual skills and attention span.

In testing for language skills, the patient might be asked to name some objects from a picture. Conceptualization is tested by the interpretation of metaphors and proverbs, while vision skills are tested by copying geometric shapes. Attention-span tests include asking the patient to count or spell forward and then backward.

It is often asked if a CAT scan or magnetic resonance imaging (MRI) of the head is necessary for the diagnosis of dementia? The answer is "no". These tests merely exclude other causes of memory loss such as a blood clot in the brain or a tumor. Certain blood tests would be done to exclude reversible causes of dementia such as Vitamin B-12 deficiency, hypothyroidism and syphilis.

There is a promising new blood test that determines what type of chromosome you have, and it may predict your chances of developing Alzheimer's disease. Apolilipoprotein E, a cholesterol-carrier protein, has been linked with Alzheimer's disease, and the gene for this protein is found on chromosome 19. Inheritance of the E4 allele of this gene indicates a substantially increased risk of Alzheimer's disease. This test is not routinely recommended for every man in the street, but it may be useful if you are suffering from memory loss and have a strong family history of Alzheimer's disease.

Estrogens & and the link to memory loss

There are multiple factors that contribute to the etiology of Alzheimer's disease. Identifying these risk factors may help us understand the entity better and in turn target preventive or curative strategies. It has been well known that family

history, Down's syndrome, head injury and thyroid disease
may increase the odds of developing dementia. Data from a
study on nuns also suggest that cerebral vascular disease
increases the risk of Alzheimer's disease in elderly women.
More recently, there have been hypotheses of a hormonal
link to Alzheimer's disease both in elderly women and men.
The elderly female has been well researched and there is
increasing evidence of a link between estrogens and
cognition. Although the Andropause, the male equivalent of
Menopause, is also associated with some decline in cognitive
function, there is relatively less data linking cognitive
changes and hormones in the elderly male. There are
several possible reasons for the effect of estrogens on
cognition:

1) It has been shown that estrogens can improve blood
   flow to diseased blood vessels, although the
   mechanism of this is not clear. Thus, in the
   postmenopausal stage, there is diminished blood flow
   to the brain, which in turn may affect cognitive
   processing.

2) Estrogens can have a direct effect on neuronal
   function and also in the repair of neurons damaged
   by disease processes. For example, estrogens have
   been shown to promote the growth of cholinergic
   neurons that are frequently damaged in Alzheimer's
   disease.

3) Apo E and amyloid deposition in the brain have been
   shown to decrease with estrogen replacement. ApoE
   and amyloid are involved in the pathogenesis of

Alzheimer's disease through development of
neurofibrillary tangles in the brain, the characteristic
pathological change seen in Alzheimer's disease.
4) The effect of estrogens on cognition may be indirect.
Estrogens interact with neurotrophins and
neurotransmitters and may modulate synaptic
plasticity, which in turn may alter cognition.

These effects on cognition by estrogens should be
considered as gradual onset modifying factors and not the
primary cause of Alzheimer's disease. In any event, most
researchers agree that the lack of estrogens does not cause
immediate decline in cognitive function. In female rats that
have had the ovaries removed (castrated), cognitive decline
did not become significant till 28 weeks after castration,
which translates to approximately 2 decades of human life.
Thus, Alzheimer's disease is not common within the first 2
decades after the menopause, but usually occurs after the
third decade.

Studies on estrogens and cognition

For more than 40 years, it has been known that the
menopause affects the health of women. Some of the
adverse health effects of menopause, such as osteoporosis
and cardiovascular disease, have been well researched and
documented. In addition, the aforesaid diseases associated
with menopause are often medically treated more
aggressively than others, such as cognitive or mood

changes. But with increasing life expectancy, women of today have to face the added challenge of cognitive decline after the menopause, secondary to the estrogen deficient state. Prominent studies, both retrospective and prospective, have revealed much of the role of estrogens in cognition.

In a retrospective study on 143 elderly female patients, researchers found that the demented group was less likely to have received estrogen replacement, compared to the non-demented group. The demented group also tended to weigh less than the non- demented group, and had a greater rate of cardiovascular disease and hip fracture. This was all attributed to the lower estrogen status of the demented patient. Another study looked at estrogen replacement and the rates of associated ischemic vascular dementia and Alzheimer's dementia in 213 women. Again, results of this study indicated that the women with dementia were less likely to have had estrogen replacement, when compared to the non-demented women. In other words, lack of estrogen replacement therapy among postmenopausal women was associated with increased likelihood of cognitive impairments, of both Alzheimer's disease and ischemic vascular dementia. This suggests that estrogen replacement therapy may well be a protective agent against dementia.

The Baltimore Longitudinal Study on Aging, a prospective multi-disciplinary study of normal aging conducted by the Institute of Aging also supports the protective influences of estrogen replacement therapy. Four hundred and seventy two post- or peri-menopausal women were followed up for 16 years. After adjusting for education, the relative risk for Alzheimer's disease in estrogen users as compared to non-users was 0.46 (95% C.I., 0.209- 0.997). This indicates a reduced risk of almost half for women who reported the use of estrogens, compared to non-users. The authors of this study hypothesized possible explanations of the protective mechanism including neurotransmitter activity, an antioxidant effect and inhibition of apolipoprotein levels in plasma.

In another study, 1124 elderly women of a New York City community center were followed prospectively. These women were not suffering from Alzheimer's disease at the start of the study. It was found through annual assessments that women who took estrogen after menopause had a much later onset of Alzheimer Disease, compared to those not on estrogen replacement therapy. One important finding from this study was that estrogen use does not seem to prevent Alzheimer's disease, but rather it delays the onset. Those using estrogen for more than one year had a significant reduction in risk of Alzheimer's disease.

A larger study involving 8877 women of Laguna Hills, California also found that the increase in Alzheimer disease in older women might be due to estrogen deficiency. The investigators reviewed the stated cause of death on the death certificates, and correlating this with whether that woman had previously been on estrogens. At the start of this study in 1981, none of the women had dementia, and all had to complete a health survey questionnaire. Of the 3760 subjects who died between 1981 and 1995, 248 women had the diagnosis of Alzheimer's disease documented in their death certificates. By analyzing the data the investigators found that the risk of Alzheimer's and related dementias was less for estrogen users than non-users (odds ratio, 0.65; 95% confidence interval 0.49- 0.88).

Henderson and his group at the University of Southern California made an interesting observation. They studied cognitive skills associated with estrogen replacement in women with Alzheimer's disease. Women on estrogen replacement were matched with non-users and men suffering from Alzheimer's disease. Their findings demonstrated that women on estrogen performed better in cognitive skills, especially in naming, verbal short-term memory and a drawing test. Their findings support the hypothesis that estrogen therapy for women with Alzheimer's disease is associated with better cognitive skills and that gender differences in Alzheimer's disease may reflect a state of acquired estrogen deficiency among women with this disorder.

Medical researchers in Japan demonstrated the benefit of estrogen use in seven specific cases. They initiated estrogen treatment in 7 women who demonstrated increasing dementia over the previous five years. Four of the seven women had marked improvement in their cognition scores on the Mini Mental Status Examination (MMSE) and the Hasegawa Dementia Scale (HDS). Two had moderate improvement and one showed no response to estrogen treatment. This study unfortunately lacked scientific credibility as the design was observational, and not placebo-controlled nor were the patients randomized. In any event, the numbers in this study were very small, and thus it is difficult to come to any concrete conclusion.

Mulnard and his group at the University of California Irvine studied the effects of estrogen replacement in 120 demented women over a 4 year period and found that estrogen therapy after one year did not improve cognitive function. The results were published in a Feb 2000 issue of the Journal of the American Medical Association. However, if the researchers had used more specific cognitive domain testing for older patients, the results may have been different, favoring positive results with estrogen therapy.

Does estrogen replacement prevent neuro-degeneration? The data from both basic sciences and clinical studies suggest it does. Although family history and age are the biggest factors in the occurrence of Alzheimer's disease, estrogen replacement therapy has demonstrated beneficial effects on cognition and mood. In the absence of absolute contraindications, physicians should consider estrogen replacement for their female patients to reduce the problems associated with an estrogen-depleted state. There has been abundant data on the benefits of estrogen replacement for osteoporosis and heart disease. Now, there appears to be the additional benefit of estrogens on cognition. The benefits have to be considered long-term and weighed against the risk, albeit small' of estrogen-dependent tumors. More prospective randomized controlled trials involving larger numbers are needed to confirm the association of estrogen replacement and Alzheimer's.

What about the male hormone Testosterone and memory loss?

I have many anecdotal reports from patients of mine without dementia who swear that their memory improved after testosterone replacement. Although I have not performed clinical studies on the effects of testosterone on men with normal cognition, I believe that the reported effect is true. A study performed in Portland, Oregon by Dr. Janowsky and his colleagues demonstrated this. The authors of this study believe that testosterone plays a role in the organization of behavior during development. In a double blind manner, they studied the verbal and visual memory, spatial cognition, motor speed, cognitive flexibility and mood of a group of healthy older men who were given testosterone for 3 months. The increase in testosterone to levels of 150% of baseline produced significant enhancement of spatial cognition, but not in other cognitive domains. This group believed that the memory effects were indirect, possibly from the conversion of testosterone to estrogens.

One of my studies, detailed later in the chapter, had findings which paralleled the above study. I also found enhancement of spatial-cognitive function, not in normal elderly men, but those suffering from dementia. My study went on beyond 3 months and only one patient developed a side effect from testosterone treatment, and that was hyper sexuality. Although his cognition improved, the treatment was stopped for obvious reasons - he became too disruptive!

85

Animal studies performed by a group at Dartmouth University revealed that androgens given to rats did not hinder hippocampal spatial memory nor were brain cells destroyed. Memory was tested in rats by the use of water mazes.

In summary, there is some support in the scientific literature for the possible role of testosterone in memory enhancement but it is scanty at the moment, especially in comparison to the work on estrogens and cognition.

My research on improving memory with Testosterone in dementia during the Andropause

I studied the hypothesis that testosterone replacement in elderly hypogonadic males (that is, those with low testosterone levels) would improve cognition, in particular visual-spatial.

The pilot study was single blind and interventional in design. Eighteen male patients with a diagnosis of dementia had their testosterone levels measured. Five patients of the 18 (28%) were deemed biochemically hypogonadic (testosterone level < 240 ng/dL). Initial MMSE (a measure of cognitive function or memory) ranged from 17 to 22. The Clock Drawing Test (CDT), being a good measure of visual-spatial abilities was used. A normal PSA level was essential before treatments. PSA is a screening test for prostate cancer and normal levels suggest absence of prostate cancer. These 4 tests that were done at baseline (serum testosterone, MMSE, CDT and serum PSA) were repeated after 3, 6 and 9 months of treatment with testosterone 200 mg, given intramuscularly.

The results I obtained were baseline mean testosterone=126.4 ng/dl, MMSE=19.4, CDT=2.2 and PSA=0.98. After 9 months of treatment, the mean testosterone level increased in the 5 patients from 126.4ng/dl to 341ng/dl (p= 0.11). The mean PSA level also increased from 0.98 to 1.37 (p= 0.07). The remarkable finding was that the MMSE score, the test for cognitive function, improved from a mean of 19.4 to 23.2 (p= 0.02). The mean CDT score also improved from 2.2 to 3.2 (p = 0.03). The low "p value" indicates that the results were highly significant statistically, which is a very important feature of clinical studies. Four of the 5 patients continued treatment beyond 9 months; one was stopped because of hypersexual behavior.

This pilot study suggested that testosterone could indeed improve cognition, including visual spatial skills, in men with mild to moderate dementia. This could be due to the modulation of neurotransmitters by testosterone. There was a small rise in PSA, which is a marker for prostate cancer. This rise was thought not to be clinically significant, with the benefits to the patient outweighing the risks.

Treating memory loss in the Andropausal years: using pharmacological and non-pharmacological means

For men with memory loss and proven to have low testosterone levels, testosterone replacement maybe the appropriate treatment. However, in advanced dementia it may be too late for this treatment.

There are several other medications that may enhance memory. Most of them work by increasing brain transmitters by preventing the natural breakdown of these transmitters. These drugs are called acetylcholinesterase inhibitors, and include Aricept, Tacrine and Exelon at the time of writing. Another drug called Reminyl is in the pipeline. They are available only on prescription from a doctor.

Although we humans need oxygen to live, paradoxically oxygen can also disrupt critical cellular processes in the body. Free oxygen radicals can damage cells, including brain cells, and lead to memory loss. Certain nutrients called antioxidants like Vitamin A, C and E, and selenium can prevent cellular damage and thereby retard memory loss during the Andropause.

The Gingko Biloba tree apparently is the oldest surviving species of trees on earth. An extract from this tree may be helpful in retarding the ravages of aging including memory loss. Medical interest in gingko stems from the herb's ability to interfere with the action of platelet activation factor (PAF), a substance that the body produces. By inhibiting PAF, gingko has been shown to retard some of the processes of aging.

There may be other means of improving memory without the use of medications. For instance, jotting down important facts that you might forget will help. It is natural for all of us to forget some details some of the time, and we need memory-aids like pieces of paper, notebooks and alarm clocks. In the andropausal years, memory loss may be more marked and using more of such tools may help. Another valuable tool for memory enhancement is the use of associations. For instance, you meet a person and he tells you his name. One way of remembering is to think of something humorous in connection with his name. Let's say you meet Charles King. You could form an image of him with a crown on his head, and consider him "royalty". The next time you meet him, he will be impressed at you recalling his name so accurately, but may be puzzled that you keep glancing on top of his head for "the crown"!

During the Andropause, one struggles to keep one's memory as sharp as a needle. Hormones and other medications are helpful some of the times, whereas adaptive techniques are better at other times.

Chapter 5:
The Psychological Impact of Aging on Sexuality

by Samer Z. Nasr M.D. & Robert S. Tan M.D.

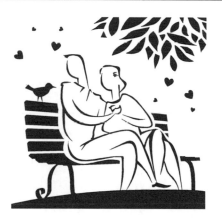

Stereotypes

We have both observed two common stereotypes about sexuality and aging in men in the so-called "Western societies", and this is especially apparent in the North American society. The male teenager is usually portrayed as a puberty driven, sexually obsessed, reckless and promiscuous individual constantly chasing young thin pretty girls and engaging in high risk sexual behavior. On the other hand, the elderly man is often seen as a weak white-haired being with no or little sex drive, cautious, monogamous and expressing his sexual feelings by harmless affectionate looks, hugs and kisses only. Of course both portrayals are highly exaggerated, but it is interesting to see that people of all age groups believe that this is the way that men should act at those stages of their life.

Aging and Sexlessness

There are many reasons why aging is associated with sexlessness. An obvious one is because Love, Sex and Romance tend to be linked with Youth. This is seen in all forms of media, from the books and magazines we read, to the television shows and movies we watch, to the playhouses and museums we patronize. How often have you seen a nude painting or sculpture of an older man? How many hit movies have portrayed a passionate romance between an elderly man and an elderly woman? How many elderly models have you seen on the front page of Elle, Vogue or Cosmopolitan? A more subtle reason for the aging-sexlessness mindset is the equation of sexuality with procreation. With elderly couples having little, if any prospects of having babies, sexual intercourse is not deemed as justifiable. While an elderly man having a much younger wife is relatively acceptable socially, that same elderly man having children as old as his existing children or great grandchildren raises many eyebrows in disapproval.

The most important reason for the association of aging and sexlessness, is the prevalent attitude that it is just not quite acceptable for older people to have sexual needs. As an experiment, just take a few moments and imagine in your own mind two very elderly individuals you personally know, totally naked and having passionate wild sex. If this makes you feel uncomfortable, there is no need to worry. Most people, young and old feel exactly the same way. This widespread denial of sexual expression in the elderly is at the origin of much of the confusion about aging and sexuality, and is contributing to many of the anxiety and depressive symptoms in older people.

Sexual desire in the Elderly

An area of widespread ignorance about sexual functioning in old age is sexual desire. Contrary to common belief, the need for sexual satisfaction and expression does not disappear with increased age. In interviewing patients in our geriatric clinics, we always include questions about sexuality. As we gained experience, we veered away from the casual and vague "everything working OK down there?" question that only a few physicians bother to ask, to very specific enquiries about frequency of intercourse, quality of erections, availability of partners and expectations (Please refer to the 15-ED in Chapter 6). Although the responses vary widely between individuals, the vast majority, both male and female, has expressed the desire to resume, improve or continue having sexual intercourse until their later years. However, despite this common desire, most still assume that total loss of sexual function is a normal part of aging. This general belief is not confirmed by research which shows that although there is a gradual decline in performance with advancing age, many people remain sexually active in their eighties and even later. One survey of people between 80 and 102 years of age showed that 88% of men and 72% of women fantasized about sex.

Let us review the main factors influencing sexuality in the later years. Many studies have shown a strong correlation between the levels of sexual activity during adulthood and sexual activity in later years. To put it simply, if you have a strong interest in sex during your youth, you will maintain that interest when you are old. Another factor influencing sexual activity in later years can be summarized by the colloquial "Use it or lose it!" People who continue to be sexually active (even by masturbating) throughout their life will experience lesser decline in sexual function as they age. But by far the most important factor impacting sexuality in later years is health. Poor health and illnesses are extremely common in the elderly. Chronic diseases such as degenerative joint disease, cardiovascular disease and diabetes are not only more prevalent in the elderly but their resulting morbidity is more severe with increasing age.

Lifestyle related behaviors such as obesity, tobacco use, lack of exercise, poor nutrition also have a greater impact on health in the elderly than at any other stage of life. This increase with age of disease burden is the main contributor to the frailty, disabilities and handicaps that are so often observed in the aged population. This in turn interferes with functioning including sexual function. For individuals in long-term relationships, the limitations caused by the poor health of one person will affect the sexual expression of their partner. The loss of a long time partner by death or divorce can also have a devastating impact on sexuality but studies have shown that many older adults remain interested in sexuality even if they lose their partner. Masturbation is also a common avenue of sexual release in the elderly who have lost a partner and are unable to find a new one. Contrary to common belief, the elderly (especially male elderly) are much more accepting of masturbation as a natural a form of sexual release than younger people.

Sexual behavior changes with Age

There is a great need to dispel some of the myths about altered sexual responses that accompany the aging process. We have seen these myths having such an oppressive impact on some of our older patients that they have openly told us that life would not be worth living anymore, and that they would seriously consider committing suicide, if their sex life came to an abrupt halt. We found the fear of impotence was so great in some populations that the mere mention that a medication may cause impotence will often result in refusal to take it. Physicians should always be very cautious about discussing the sexual side effects of medications.

Concerned health care givers should always discuss in detail the frequently unasked questions, those that we get to hear only after WE bring up the topic of sexuality. Common ones are: "What are the chances that it will affect me/my performance?" "What should I look for?" "Do I really need to take this medication?" "Can you give me another one that will not affect me in that way?" And the most frequent statement of all, "I am already having a tough time having sex as it is. I really do not want to make it worse!"

Most of the changes with age affect the intensity and duration of the four phases of the sexual response cycle. *The excitement phase* lengthens considerably: instead of the few seconds many young male need to experience an erection, older men require several minutes of stimulation before being able to achieve an erection. Direct physical stimulation such as hand caressing or oral stimulation is often needed. This is the first sign of sexual changes that is noticed by aging men and it often causes alarm and fear of impotence. It is essential to understand that this delayed erection time is normal and that this alteration will have very little effect on their actual enjoyment. Otherwise, the anxiety and the preoccupation may be such that the fear becomes a reality. *The plateau phase* also lengthens and the testes will not elevate as much as in the elderly. Complete erection is delayed often until just before orgasm. These changes can actually perceived be perceived as an advantage. Older men can sustain the plateau phase much longer and have greater ejaculatory control, thus having a prolonged opportunity to satisfy their partners and enjoy other sensations besides ejaculation. *The orgasm phase* remains present in the majority of men but its intensity declines with age. The most frequent manifestation is the absence of ejaculatory inevitability (the sensation of reaching a point where ejaculation cannot be delayed anymore). Other manifestations include a reduction in the number of muscular contractions during ejaculation and a decreased expulsion force expulsion. The ejaculate fluid is also thinner and in smaller quantity. *The resolution phase* is faster in older men, the loss of erection is more rapid and the testicles descend immediately after ejaculation. The refractory period between orgasm and the next excitement phase gradually lengthens with age starting in the mid-thirties and lasting for several hours by the sixties. It is not uncommon for that refractory period to last days in some cases.

It is important for men to realize these physiological changes that can happen to their bodies as they age. Not only is it important to realize this, but it is essential that their partners understand this as well. This will lead to less misunderstanding, and dispel myths about unattractiveness of the other partner.

Relationships changes with Age

As you get older, you actually have more time to enjoy each other. You may find that there are more opportunities for sexual expression. Older people may have less intercourse because of concomitant illnesses, but the intimacy is actually increased. It is quality rather than quantity as one ages. Enjoyment of sex does not decline but there may be need for changes in sexual techniques. During the Andropause and Menopause, there is also freedom from contraception and the worry of pregnancy. Alternative sexual expressions have to be learnt. Sexual interest in the partner undergoes a different dimension.

Androgyny in later life

The Andropause and the Menopause may bring about gender role changes. Males become less dominant, and take on a more feminine role. They prefer to be at home, tend to their yard or the grandchildren. Women on the other hand feel that this is the time to catch up. Many take on new careers, go back to school or become publicly and socially more active.

As such, gender role differences diminish. Males and females who are beyond the Andropause and Menopause may take on opposite roles. Men become less dominant and women more dominant, and this often results in blurring of the sexes.

At the same time, men's emotional expressiveness is increased. Andropausal men suddenly recall birthdays, are more into festivities and less focused on issues of business, power and wealth. However, the increased assertiveness of older women can get in the way, and this can result in marital discord with frequent arguments and fights. The lack of testosterone in older men and estrogens in older women may lead to psychological changes that impact not only their physical but mental health. This power shift in the marital relationship can lead to depression, hopelessness and at times even suicide for some. This is a frequently neglected health topic, and many physicians are not trained to recognize these changes.

Tips to lead healthy post Andropausal and Menopausal years

More will be discussed in the final chapter, but these are important tips from both of us. In combination, we have managed thousands of older men and women and wish to share some secrets of their successes.

- Regular exercise, a healthy diet and avoiding hazardous habits (smoking, alcohol excess) throughout life will contribute to general and sexual health at all ages. Even in elderly individuals with established impairments, regular physical activity and life style changes will result in an enhanced sexual desire and performance.
- It is important to educate the older man that his partner is also aging and that there are some physiological changes occurring in her too. The fall in estrogens may lead to memory loss, weakness and weakening of bones. On top of that, a woman may

have sexual difficulties from the menopause. There could be pain or discomfort during intercourse because of lack of lubrication. Estrogen replacement orally or topically can reverse some of that. There could also be diminishing desire and enjoyment of sexual activity in the aging female. This can have a negative effect on the man's sexuality and result in the older man developing sexual problems.

- Stay with your spouse during the andropausal and menopausal years. It is a growing experience and there needs to be mutual understanding. Continue to learn to adapt and help each other. Too often, we see older couples in major disagreements, and deep relationships, which were tenderly built over years, become tragically destroyed.

Chapter 6:
Hope for Men's Sexual Dysfunction

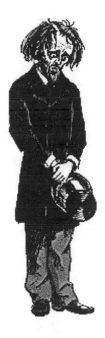

"Doctor, there is something else before I leave....I have difficulty with my nature"

This is what some men have resorted to confide in me, because they were not comfortable making direct references to the genitals. Men are, by and large, embarrassed to admit impotence, as it is viewed as the loss of manhood. Quite typically, impotence is the last issue a patient brings up just before leaving the room, almost as if he needed to build up courage before mentioning it. When dealing with a very private matter such as impotence, it does not help to have a nurse interview the patient before seeing the doctor because rarely is this problem verbalized to her.

What is sexual function and dysfunction?

Normal sexual function is much more than being able to have a penile erection or an ejaculation. There is also the dimension of libido, the feeling of desire, drive and energy associated with sexual stimulus. It is very possible to have an erection that is not accompanied by increased libido. In fact some disease states can lead to what we call a "pathological erection" - an abnormal erection that occurs in the absence of any sexual stimulus. For example, in sickle cell anemia, abnormally shaped blood cells can get sluggish and be trapped in the blood vessels of the penis, resulting in an abnormal erection. In fact this is a very painful erection, almost tormenting, and the condition is called priapism. Priapism can also be a rare side effect of a medication called trazodone, commonly used to treat depression and insomnia.

Mr. B.D.

I have often observed that paralyzed patients can have quite normal libido, but not have the ability to have an erection. Mr. B.D. was a patient of mine who exemplified this. He was a 50 year-old man living in a nursing home, paralyzed from the waist down because of a motor vehicle accident. His spinal cord was damaged resulting in the loss of bladder, bowel function and the use of his legs. Yet he was always preoccupied with his sexual fantasies, often imagining dates with women from out of state. Below the seat of his wheelchair, you could often find the latest issue of a magazine such as Playboy, often to the horror of nurses attending to him! Mr. BD had very normal libido, despite the inability to have an erection or an ejaculation as a result of his accident.

Aging results in a decline in sexual function. Part of the reason could be the loss of nerve cells in the brain areas that process pleasurable feelings. Also, the sense of touch is diminished and could result in lowering of libido. As one gets old, the likelihood of arteriosclerosis and diabetes increase, all serving to decrease blood flow to the penis and resulting in erectile dysfunction. The force of ejaculation, amount of ejaculate, the time required to achieve an erection are all decreased with the aging process.

Normal male sexual response has four major phases - desire, arousal (erection), orgasm and relaxation. There can be disorders at various states. Erection is the most common phase which men have difficulty with when they complain of sexual dysfunction.

Impotence is nowadays more frequently referred to as "erectile dysfunction", which is defined as "the persistent inability to attain or maintain penile erection sufficient for sexual intercourse". In 1992, the National Institute of Health

Consensus Development Conference recommended the term "erectile dysfunction" as it more accurately defines the problem and may have less disparaging connotations. It is estimated that in America 20 to 30 million men have some degree of erectile dysfunction.

With the introduction of newer drugs like Viagra, further bolstered by the accompanying media hype, patients are becoming increasingly more open about this medical problem, and erectile dysfunction is being presented more and more frequently for medical attention. In reality, erectile dysfunction occurs most commonly as part and parcel of Andropause. However, getting treatment is still a long crusade, as some managed care companies do not reimburse for erectile dysfunction medications, as it is not considered by some to be an illness, unlike diabetes or high blood pressure. Thankfully, politicians like Bob Dole have come up and publicly declared that their problem with erectile dysfunction, and how it can be reversed with adequate treatment. Slowly, but surely, the Andropause and the related symptom of erectile dysfunction will be more widely accepted, and men will no longer have to suffer in silence.

Anatomy of the penis – knowing thy parts

The penis consists of two parallel cylindrical tissues called the corpora cavernosa (B). There is also a smaller single cylinder called corpus spongiosum (C) which surrounds the urethra (D), the tube where urine passes out. To simplify it, you can consider the penis as a 3 cylinder engine - doesn't sound much in terms of horsepower but it does it's job when it is properly tuned up! The corpora cavernosa (B) are composed of a network of interconnected spaces, and blood flows freely in these spaces. Blood from these spaces drain into post-cavernous venules that join up to become the large emissary veins. These then ultimately join together to become the deep dorsal vein (A) as illustrated in Figure 3.

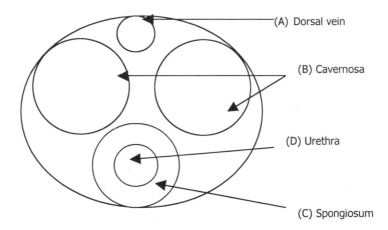

Figure 3: Cross- section of penis

Both autonomic as well as somatic nerves supply the penis. Parasympathethic nerves come form the sacral segments in the spinal cord, while sympathetic nerves come form the lower thoracic and upper lumbar segments. Somatic sensory and motor fibers enter and leave the sacral cord and innervate the penis by the pudendal nerve. As a result of the anatomical disposition of the nerves, it is no surprise that patient with spinal cord injury loose their ability to have an erection.

Physiology of erection - how it works

While the penis is flaccid or in a natural resting state, there is a balance of blood flow in and out of the 3 cylinders mentioned above. To obtain an erection, interaction between the nerves and blood vessels is essential, caused by both a central psychogenic stimulus as well as a reflexogenic mechanism. Psychogenic erections occur when a person is stimulated either by sound, smell or sight - what we call the senses. Reflexogenic erections result form touching the penis and activating sensory receptors.

When a man is sexually aroused, the *parasympathetic system* is activated and triggers a series of events starting with the release of *nitric oxide* and ends up with increased levels of cyclic guanosine monophosphate (cGMP). Nitric oxide is similar to laughing gas, so we can call it the "pleasure substance". In fact the drug Viagra works in part by enhancing nitrous oxide. The increase in cGMP causes the blood vessels and muscles in the penis to relax initially, allowing it to fill with blood. As a consequence, the 3 cylinders fill up and swell. The rapid filling of the cylinders also compress the venules and prevents the blood from escaping out of the cavernous spaces, causing a more rigid state. The result is that an erection occurs.

Classifying erectile dysfunction

Erectile dysfunction is probably the most significant symptom in andropausal men, but it may or may not be the sentinel event of the Andropause. This is because there are many reversible causes of erectile dysfunction that may be related to disease states.

Some cases of erectile dysfunction are psychogenic and others are organic. At one time, doctors assumed that most cases of erectile dysfunction were psychogenic, but today we believe that up to 80% can be organic. We used to think a person was impotent because of anxiety, stress and the like. With the introduction of Viagra, and a better the understanding of the Andropause, we now view organic causes as predominant.

What can predispose me to erectile dysfunction?

a) Hormones

In the Andropause, testosterone levels drop and 25% of older men are hypogonadic. In the medical literature, there is controversy as to whether the lack of hormones such as testosterone causes erectile dysfunction. Some doctors dismiss the idea that testosterone deficiency can be a cause of erectile dysfunction. My belief is that testosterone improves erectile dysfunction in older men especially when they are hypogonadic, and many patients of mine have demonstrated improvements of erectile dysfunction with testosterone treatment. In particular, many have told me that their spontaneous nighttime erections improve. The improvement in erectile dysfunction with testosterone administration could be a direct effect on the testosterone receptors, the improvement of libido (a central effect), a general improvement in well-being or an increase in muscle strength. In younger men, with normal testosterone levels, there is little role in using testosterone to boost sexual prowess.

b) **Psychogenic**

There is a strong relationship between erectile dysfunction and depression. Many men who suffer from depression also have erectile dysfunction. The situation may be like the chicken-and-egg analogy, in that depression can cause erectile dysfunction, and conversely, erectile dysfunction can cause depression. The treatment of depression with antidepressants can improve erectile dysfunction, and likewise, treatment of erectile dysfunction can result in improvements in moods.

The Massachusetts Male Aging Study is probably the largest database on the issues of male aging, including impotence. This study, conducted by the New England Research Institute, has been going on for years. In one of their analyses reported in a 1998 issue of Psychosomatic Medicine, it was found that depression was 1.8 times more common in patients who reported erectile dysfunction. This was independent of confounding factors such as lifestyle factors, health status, medication use and hormones.

Mr. A.N.

Mr. A.N. was a 65 year-old business executive, always rushing around and complaining. He had multiple medical problems, including high blood pressure, high cholesterol and a bad back. He always appeared stressed and tired, and honestly he looked depressed to me. At the next consultation, I administered a test called the Geriatric Depression Scale on him. I wasn't surprised at the result, which indicated he was clinically depressed. I started exploring issues with him, and he confessed that his wife was complaining of his inability to perform sexually. Examination revealed that he was well virilized and had normal sized testicles. True enough, his testosterone level came back as normal. I started him on Viagra, as well as an antidepressant called Zoloft. Four weeks later, he came back to me a changed man, feeling so much better that he seemingly forgot about his blood pressure and cholesterol problems. This was a situation where treatment with testosterone had not seemed appropriate.

c) Vascular (Blood vessels)

If you have high blood pressure, cholesterol problems, diabetes or smoke too much, the arterial blood vessels in the cylinders of the penis could be damaged. Blood flow is minimized, because the blood vessels cannot fill adequately with blood. If the blood vessels of the veins do not close to trap blood in the cavernous spaces, this can lead to erectile dysfunction. Drugs that act on blood vessels such as Viagra act by allowing the blood vessels to relax and fill with blood.

d) **Drugs**

Several drugs have been implicated to cause erectile dysfunction. Certain drugs commonly used to treat psychosis, depression and high blood pressure can affect neurotransmitter chemicals such as serotonin, adrenalin and noradrenalin. Examples include haldoperidol (Haldol), amitriptyline (Elavil) and methyldopa (Aldomet). Beta-blockers such as propranolol (Inderal) cause erectile dysfunction by potentiating alpha-adrenergic activities in the penis, thereby helping to drain the blood in the penis (please refer to the section on the physiology of erection). Certain "water pills" such as thiazide diuretics and spironolactone (Aldactone) can cause erectile dysfunction, although the mechanism is unclear.

Cimetidine (Tagamet) is known to decrease libido and cause erectile dysfunction by acting against androgens like testosterone. It may even cause your breast to swell, a condition called gynaecomastia. When treating stomach ulcers today, I would recommend avoiding this drug if at all possible as there are much better newer drugs. Estrogens are sometimes used by men to treat prostate cancer and certainly can be a cause of erectile dysfunction. An antifungal drug called ketoconazole (Nizoral) is another culprit.

e) **Smoking and Alcohol**

Smoking causes blood vessels in the penis to constrict and thus decreases blood flow to the penis. Alcohol in small amounts improves erection and may increase libido but large amounts of consumption can lead to erectile dysfunction. If alcohol is consumed in excess, it can also suppress testosterone production, which may lead to decreased libido and subsequent erectile dysfunction. My research on smoking and the Andropause suggest that smoking per se may lead to decreased testosterone and hence an earlier Andropause.

f) **Chronic illnesses**

If you are ill and unwell, suffering from a chronic condition like diabetes, kidney failure, heart failure, arteriosclerosis, you are more likely to be having erectile dysfunction. There are studies that have found that 50% of men with chronic diabetes have erectile dysfunction. Diabetes is a disease that results from high blood sugar. What a lot of people do not realize is that high blood sugar levels attack your blood vessels, both big and small. Eventually, as the blood vessels are destroyed less blood is able to flow to the penis, resulting in erectile dysfunction.

g) Nerve causes

Nerve disorders such as Parkinson's disease, Alzheimer's disease, stroke and head injury often cause erectile dysfunction by decreasing libido or preventing the initiation of an erection. Spinal cord lesions from an accident may also cause this effect. The sense of touch, which is mediated through transmission of nerves, is also diminished with aging, and the penis becomes less sensitive to touch, leading to problems with erection.

What does the doctor look for?

When you see your doctor, be as honest as you can, as this will help him help you. The other important task is to identify a doctor who is sympathetic towards you and knows how to treat such illnesses. Do you need to see a specialist? That really depends on the health insurance plan you are on, and also the training of your primary care doctor. By and large, primary care physicians like internists and family physicians are adequate. A specialist who can help you could be a Geriatrician like myself, or an Urologist.

The doctor you see will probe you on some very private questions. Don't be embarrassed, particularly if you have the erectile dysfunction – openly tell him or her. If you are under tremendous stress, let it be known. Do not hide your drinking or smoking history. List all the medical conditions you have, and bring all the medicines you take. Be comfortable with your own anatomy, and differentiate in your mind if have sexual desire but cannot have an erection, or you do not have any desire at all! Your doctor needs to know if you have pure erectile dysfunction or libido issues.

The following questionnaire, termed the 15-ED may be a helpful starting point. Answer it and bring it along when you see your doctor.

The 15 item Erectile Dysfunction (The 15-ED ©) Questionnaire, by R Tan MD

---

1. At what age did this problem start?
2. Was it associated with a specific event?
3. Did it come on gradually or all of a sudden?
4. Do you get a partial erection, and if so how many percent?
5. How often in a week do you have this problem?
6. Is there an erection when you sleep or dream?
7. Does the problem occur with some partners or all partners?
8. Do you have a problem producing seminal fluid?
9. What illnesses do you suffer from?
10. What drugs are you taking?
11. Do you use recreational drugs like cocaine?
12. Do you smoke? How much?
13. Do you drink? How much?
14. Is there stress in your life?
15. How are you getting along with your partner?

At some point, your doctor is going to examine you, so be prepared! Apart from a general examination, the doctor will be pay particular attention to your circulatory and neurological systems. Your genitals will be inspected and the doctor will be on the lookout for hypospadias (spilt penis), phimosis (tight foreskin) and signs of hypogonadism (low testosterone). Hypogonadic signs include loss of hair and small testicular size. The size of the resting penis will be determined, but there is a wide range, and may vary from culture to culture. Generally speaking, it is 3.5 to 5 cm long in the resting or unaroused stage. The doctor may also perform a rectal examination to check your prostate.

Blood tests may be performed and typically the blood levels of testosterone, prolactin (to exclude a rare brain tumor), FSH and LH will be obtained. A PSA level may be performed by your physician if he is contemplating treating you with testosterone. An EKG (heart tracing) may be done if you are to begin treatment with Viagra.

In more complex cases, a test called nocturnal penile tumescence and an injection of a prostaglandin into the penis may be performed. This may help the doctor determine if the cause of your erectile dysfunction to be either vascular or neurogenic in origin. These tests are not routinely necessary and reserved for cases that need further evaluation.

What treatments are available?

It was not too long ago when very little was available for the treatment of erectile dysfunction. Fortunately, over the last 10 years, there have been many advances and I believe there are even more on the horizon.

a) Testosterone

Does testosterone correct erectile dysfunction? The answer is both yes and no. Scientists have argued about this for a long time. There are proponents for and against. My personal experience from clinical experience tells me that the it is more complicated than just topping up testosterone when it is low for patients suffering from erectile dysfunction. To confuse matters more, some patients of mine with erectile dysfunction have benefited from testosterone despite having normal levels.

A study was done by Johnson & Jarrow and reported in the Journal of Urology in 1992. They looked at the feasibility of endocrine screening of impotent men in an effort to identify a treatable cause of impotence. The purpose of the screening was to determine the prevalence of endocrine problems, particularly low testosterone or hypogonadism. Only 2.1% of the impotent men (7 of the 330 screened) had hypogonadism. However 5 of the 7 men who were hypogonadic had smaller testicles than those who were eugonadic (normal testosterone level). The authors of this study suggested that screening for hypogonadism would only be cost effective if a careful examination was carried out prior to doing any blood tests, to identify those with small testicles. My personal experience working with an older population suggests that the prevalence rate of hypogonadism in patients who complain of impotence is actually higher. About 1 in 4 of older patients have hypogonadism as a cause of their erectile dysfunction.

The testosterone story remains a bit of a mystery. Recently, some Italian investigators reported in the International Journal of Andrology that regardless of the cause of erectile dysfunction, the outcome of treatment, either with testosterone or non-testosterone substances, raised the blood levels of testosterone. Non-testosterone treatments to correct impotence include nitrous oxide vasodilators (blood vessel expanders) like Viagra, prostaglandins like Caverject and MUSE. The findings of this study suggests to me that the body is capable of producing increased amounts of testosterone, and that there are many ways to correct impotence through raising the body's production of testosterone.

How important is testosterone in establishing sexuality in men? An interesting paper published in the Journal Clinical Endocrinology and Metabolism in 1982 tried to illustrate this. There have been studies that demonstrate a positive dose-response relationship between testosterone levels and sexual performance. However, other studies have also demonstrated that many aspects of sexual function are maintained despite having testosterone levels that are well below normal. Why this is so is unclear. Nevertheless, in normal populations, high levels of testosterone are correlated with more vigorous responses to visual erotic stimuli. Although testosterone declines during aging parallel the decline in sexual function, hormonal changes contribute to perhaps only a minor extent compared to behavioral changes. The initial action of testosterone may be on libido factors, which in turn lead to stimulation of other aspects of sexuality. According to the authors, testosterone could act by stimulating genital sensations and enhancing other pleasurable awareness of the sexual response, rather than directly affecting the brain in the promotion of sexual imagery.

In a study on hypogonadic men reported in the Journal of Clinical Endocrinology and Metabolism in 1983, the authors found that the erectile responses to erotic films and fantasy were not lower in hypogonadic patients as compared to normal men. Paradoxically, after erection, some of the hypogonadic men took a longer time for the penis to return to normal size. However, spontaneous erections, both during sleep and waking, were less frequent in hypogonadic men. I wish to discuss a patient I saw who resumed having spontaneous erections at night after treatment with testosterone.

Mr. C.R.

Mr. C.R. was a 75 year-old man crippled with severe arthritis, high blood pressure and diabetes. He looked tired and typified a patient that "had lost his manhood"!
On examination, his arm pits revealed no hair, his testicles were shriveled, and his skin was dry. I was not surprised when his total testosterone came back at 190 ng/dl (normal range is 241 to 827). Three days after his treatment with intramuscular testosterone, he called me to say that he was starting to have spontaneous erections. He said: "It was waking me up when I was asleep. I sure had pleasant dreams". He was beaming the next time I saw him on his follow up visit. He said his skin was less dry and that he was a much happier man.

What do I personally think of testosterone and hypo-sexuality? I do not believe that testosterone replacement will restore sexuality in everyone. In my experience, I have found testosterone to work 80% of the time for those who were impotent and had low testosterone levels. By and large, for those with normal testosterone, I have found that the role of testosterone is limited. In this group of patients who are not hypogonadic, I am more in favor of the use of drugs such as Viagra and Caverject that act on the blood vessels in the penis. Whatever the case, for testosterone to work, I believe the patient has to play his part too. Just as for body builders who use hormones, maximal benefit results when combined with intensive exercise. For patients on testosterone replacement, I would suggest a regimen of exercises for the pelvic (levator ani) muscles - a modification of Kegel exercises that many post-menopausal women do to restore urinary control.

It is my belief that testosterone plays a supplementary role in correcting erectile dysfunction. Some of this is achieved by improving libido, and some by improving general muscle strength. There are testosterone receptors in the genitals that could be stimulated not only by naturally produced testosterone, but by exogenous testosterone as well.

b) Sildenafil (Viagra)

This drug needs little introduction, having enjoyed massive publicity when it was launched into the market in 1998. In fact its sales helped the Pfizer pharmaceutical company skyrocket the value of its stock at that time. When sexual stimulation occurs, there is release of a substance called nitrous oxide into the penis muscle. The inhibition of an enzyme (phosphodiseterase) by Viagra causes a marked rise of cyclic GMP and this results in increased muscle relaxation and better erection. Viagra has no effect on the penis if there is no sexual stimulation and when the concentrations of nitrous oxide and cyclic GMP are low.

Viagra has been evaluated in more than 20 clinical trials and several hundreds of thousands of men have been on this drug in the past few years. What we know is that Viagra does not improve libido like testosterone but may be a wonderful complement to testosterone for andropausal men. The drug is by and large very safe, although some deaths have been reported with the use of Viagra. These were men who had bad coronary disease and died of a heart attack. Sexual activity is a risk factor for heart attack in less than 1% of patients. If you have heart trouble, especially if you had a recent heart attack, this drug may not be for you. Your doctor may want to do a cardiac stress test before starting you on Viagra. Some men have complained of headache, flushing, stomach problems, nasal stuffiness and abnormal vision after taking this drug. It may also cause a rare retinal disease and it is best to have your eye doctor check you over if you are worried. I must state that these side effects are rare and very few patients experience these symptoms.

The drug comes in 2 doses, 50mg and 100mg. It should be taken one hour before sexual activity. Remember it does not improve libido, and if you are taking the drug, you have to work at it too, although I would leave it to your own imagination as how to achieve that!

c) **Alprostadil (Caverject)**

Caverject works close to 70% of the time. This is a prostaglandin that you inject into the side of the penis to achieve an erection. For some, this may be a daunting task and you may need some skill and training before you can do this. The side effect can be painful erection.

Like Viagra and testosterone, it is available only by prescription.

This prostaglandin can also be inserted into your urethra, the hole where the urine comes out of the penis. You can refer to the chapter discussing the anatomy of the male genitalia. Alprostadil inserted through the urethra may seem a less daunting task than penile injection, and many men prefer this. It however is less effective than the injectable method. There are few side effects but may include pain in the penis.

d) Yohimbine

This drug is obtained from the bark of the yohim tree. It acts on adrenergic receptors in the brain and as such may help libido as well. Some men get palpitations, a fine tremor, raised blood pressure and anxiety with the use of this drug.

Drugs not yet approved by the FDA

There are some drugs that are available in other countries but not yet approved by the Food and Drug Administration (FDA) for use in the United States. This does not mean that they do not work. It could be that there is lack of funding to promote them, or it simply takes more time to get through the stringent process required by the government.

a) Papaverine

This drug works in up to 80% of men, but it does not work very well for those who have a vascular cause for their erectile dysfunction. Like Viagra it also increases cyclic GMP, but is less expensive.

b) Phentolamine (Vasomax)

This drug works about 40% of the time. It can be potentially used alone or in combination with papaverine. It has side effects of headache, facial flush and nasal stuffiness may cause the blood pressure to bottom out. The FDA is reviewing this drug's potential of brown fat accumulation in animal studies. The implication of brown fat accumulation in older males is probably not very consequential.

c) Apormorphine (Uprima)

This is a kind of morphine and acts on the dopamine receptors in the brain. An under-the-tongue preparation is being developed at the moment, and may be available in 2002 . A possible advantage of Uprima over Viagra would be faster onset of action because of quicker absorption under the tongue. Studies performed have shown it to be safe in patients with coronary artery disease and hypertension.

Mr.J.C.

A 76 year-old man, married for 30 years, Mr. J.C. came to see me supposedly for health maintenance. All he had wanted was the flu shot as it was late fall. On his way out, he looked at me sheepishly and said, "Doctor, there is something else before I leave. You know, I have been married for 30 years and we have had a happy marriage. My wife is 70 years old, and we still enjoy each other very much. But..." he started to sob, "I am afraid that I am losing it all. I have no more desire and the Mrs. is not very happy. I am afraid that she might be looking elsewhere, and I cannot blame her........."

So what was the problem? I used the 15-ED questionnaire on him, and had very telling results. He was drinking 5 beers every night, and had smoked 20 cigarettes a day for the past 40 years. Also, he was taking blood pressure medications. His erectile dysfunction has set in gradually over the past 6 months.

He had clinical signs of hypogonadism as his testicles were shrunken, and much of his pubic hair was lost. The first thing I did was to counsel him on his smoking and drinking. I then ordered some lab tests including testosterone levels, and switched his blood pressure medications.

Two weeks later, he came back, still unsatisfied. His testosterone had come back at 189 ng/dl, which was low. He was started on Androgel, and reviewed 4 weeks later. This time, he was a little happier, saying his erectile dysfunction was about 50% better. I discussed injectable Caverject and oral Viagra with him, and he made his choice between the two. After one week, he called me to say how very happy he was now.

The point I am illustrating from this case is that the treatment of erectile dysfunction requires patience from both the patient and the doctor. Some cases may not be fixed overnight, and it needs a partnership between the patient and the doctor to achieve success. It may be a dreadfully humiliating experience to admit that you have erectile dysfunction in the Andropause, but admitting it is your best way to recovery.

Chapter 7:
Testosterone Replacement in the Andropause

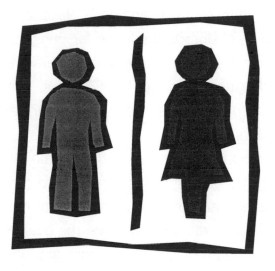

Hormones for women, why not men?

In this day and age, postmenopausal women are often prescribed estrogen replacement therapy, but testosterone replacement for elderly men is not yet routine treatment. Part of the reason is that doctors are trained with the dictum that "If you can do no good, then do no harm", which is part of the Hippocratic oath. The Food and Drug Administration (FDA) has not yet approved hormonal replacement for elderly men, and so it is left to the individual doctor to decide whether his patient should receive hormonal therapy.

It is doubtless that hormonal therapy benefits elderly men as evidenced by research. However, the general physician community remains skeptical and unenthusiastic because the basis of all treatment, as taught in medical schools, has to be "evidence based". "Evidenced based" means that large clinical trials involving thousands of men have had to be done, and comparison made against a placebo, to ensure there was no bias. Unfortunately, so far, most of the trials on testosterone replacement are small, averaging about 20 subjects, and lasting no longer than 2 years. The major reason for the small sample sizes in these clinical trials was the pitiful lack of funding.

Although much is known of the female Menopause, little research has been done with respect to the male equivalent called Andropause. In contrast to Menopause, which is a relatively rapid event when the ovaries shut down, Andropause is thought to be much more gradual process. There are many similarities, however, such as the physiological rise of follicular stimulating hormone (FSH) and luteinizing hormone (LH) associated with a decline of both estrogen and testosterone. In men however, the corresponding elevations of FSH and LH are less marked than in post-menopausal women. But it does happen! Recently, I showed some laboratory results (raised FSH & LH) to a resident in Obstetrics & Gynecology who was rotating through Geriatrics, and quizzed her on the significance of the results. She assumed that the patient was female and felt a little insulted that such a question be posed to a future OBGYN. Lo and behold, when I asked her to look at the gender written on the result sheet, her jaw dropped! She told me that this was the first time she had ever heard of the Andropause, although obviously being very familiar with the Menopause. Similarly, many of the physicians out there may not have heard about the Andropause, because they were never taught this entity. Hopefully there will be more and more sympathetic physicians who will agree to appropriate testosterone replacement in old age.

Obstacles to Testosterone replacement for Men

I have already mentioned two possible reasons why testosterone is not routinely prescribed to older men. To recapitulate, they are the lack of large clinical trials and physician apathy or ignorance.

There are additional reasons. Historically, testosterone has been a drug that has been much abused. Athletes, in the attempt to clip off a few crucial seconds and beat the record, have used testosterone and other anabolic hormones, a practice viewed in competitive sports as blatant cheating. Hence there may be a stigma when older men who are hypogonadic are prescribed testosterone. Perhaps they are criticized as cheating nature, because they refuse to accept the natural process of aging and are trying to defeat it. However, in my opinion, NOT being on testosterone when you need it is cheating yourself. It is no different from diabetics using insulin because their bodies do not produce adequate amounts naturally. In my estimate about 5 to10 million men above 65 in America are hypogonadic or low on testosterone. This is an estimation based on studies indicating a prevalence rate of hypogonadism of 25% in men above 65 years.

Molecular aspects of Testosterone

Androgens are synthesized from cholesterol and joined into four fused carbon rings. Yes, that infamous rogue cholesterol is the precursor of testosterone! Perhaps, this is the reason that seafood such as oysters, shrimp and lobsters, all of which are high in cholesterol, are thought to be aphrodisiacs. Not that I am suggesting that you sacrifice your health for the sake of love by consuming shrimps excessively!

Dehydroepiandrosterone (DHEA) is the principal androgenic steroid produced by the adrenal cortex and is a precursor of both testosterone and estradiol. Adrenal androgens have little intrinsic biologic activity and are primarily active only after conversion in the peripheral tissues to testosterone. Most effects of androgens are mediated through an androgen receptor, a 919 amino-acid protein. Once androgen is bound, active transcription occurs producing messenger RNA. Messenger RNA encodes a wide variety of enzymatic, structural and receptor proteins. It is unclear if aging affects this process, although it is known for a fact that, aging is associated with a decline in the production of DHEA. Currently, DHEA is available commercially as a non-prescription "health food" in most pharmacies and health food stores.

The history of Testosterone synthesis

From time immoral, men have created crude forms of testosterone replacement, and to this day, many Eastern cultures still practice such rituals. In China, men have consumed testicles of animals such as bulls in various concoctions. Sometimes it was prepared as a "love potion" to be drunk in a small cup. In India, the Hindu Ayervedic system of medicine promoted the consumption of testicular tissue to treat impotence. Almost 2000 years ago, the Greek physician Pliny recommended eating animal testicles to improve sexual dysfunction. The Spaniards have a delicacy called *cojones*, which is in fact, cooked bulls testicles.

Fortunately, with modern-day science and technology, we are now able to synthesize pure testosterone by chemical means, rather than relying on the extraction from animal parts. In fact, when it is consumed orally, testosterone undergoes what is called the "first pass effect", whereby most of it is destroyed by the liver, and very little testosterone ends up reaching the other parts of the body. Thus the only effective way of getting testosterone to the whole body is either through an injection, or applied to the skin through which it is absorbed. These methods of administration would enable testosterone to bypass the liver, and thus circumvent the "first pass" effect.

In chapter two, I talked about the Dr. Brown Sequard, a genius who bravely injected himself with a concoction of bull's testicles and reported the effects in the Lancet. This experiment was conducted towards the end of the 19th century, way before pharmaceutical companies figured out a synthetic preparation.

In 1935 in Amsterdam, Professor Ernst Lacquer and his team at Organon pharmaceutical company discovered synthesized a few precious crystals from a large source of bulls' testicles. In fact, he should be credited for the word testosterone, after presenting a paper called "Crystalline male hormone from testicles". To date, the Organon Company is still manufacturing testosterone, the oral form called Andriol.

Professor Adolph Butenandt, who was with Schering pharmaceutical company, synthesized a few crystals of androstenedione, a relatively inactive urinary breakdown product of testosterone. This had been diligently prepared from the urine from volunteer policemen, a quantity so much that apparently there was enough to fill an Olympic-sized swimming pool! It was a mammoth task as only 15mg of crystals were synthesized! Subsequently, he formulated the structure of testosterone and published it in 1935.

In 1935, Leopold Ruzicka, working for Ciba pharmaceutical company announced a patent on the method of production of testosterone from cholesterol around the same time as Butenandt did. For this work, both Ruzicka and Butenandt won the Nobel Prize in 1939. Yes, the discovery of testosterone was deemed significant enough for the highest award in science, the Nobel Prize!

Soon after, a slow-release form of testosterone called testosterone propionate given by injection was produced. This drug has been in use now for about 60 years, and it was not until the last 5 years that alternative delivery forms have been developed. Testoderm, a patch applied to the scrotum was followed by Androderm, a patch applied anywhere on the skin. A gel form called Androgel became available in the summer of 2000.

The administration of Testosterone

There are five different delivery forms of testosterone currently available:
1) Oral testosterone
2) Long-acting testosterone pellets, implanted under the skin
3) Short acting testosterone injection (propionate and aqueous testosterone)
4) Long-acting testosterone injection (enanthate and cypionate)
5) Transdermal testosterone systems

Use of oral testosterone is limited because of the "first pass effect" and the risk of damage to the liver. Testosterone pellets for subcutaneous implantation are not widely acceptable in elderly males. Short-acting testosterone propionate and aqueous testosterone injections are not practical for long-term use because the short duration of action would necessitate frequent dosaging throughout the day. Probably the most commonly used dosage form is long-acting testosterone esters (enanthate and cypionate) given by injections. Unfortunately the pharmacokinetic profile of these esters is problematic. Serum testosterone levels are often very high during the first few days following injection and fall to below normal at the end of the dosing interval. Although the use of weekly injections may sustain serum testosterone levels within the normal range, such frequency of injections is not acceptable to most patients. Hence the usual regimen of either testosterone cypionate or enanthate is 150 to 200 mg intramuscularly every 2 weeks. I have found that sometimes, older patients do very well with just a once-a-month dosing.

At the time of writing, topical testosterone patches were recently introduced. Skin patches are attractive because of their improved pharmacokinetic profile. Transdermal testosterone systems mimic the circadian rhythm observed in normal healthy men, and the wide fluctuations associated with testosterone injections are avoided. There are 2 topical testosterone patches currently available in the U.S. and these two differ in sites of application. One is applied to scrotal skin and the other is applied to clean dry skin of the back, abdomen, upper arms or thighs. Local reactions are the most commonly reported adverse reaction and in general, tolerability of either patch is excellent. However, cost may be the prohibitive factor for some patients.

The transdermal gel of testosterone was FDA

approved in the summer of 2000. This is a clear colorless hydro-alcoholic containing 1% testosterone and provides continuous transdermal delivery of testosterone over a 24-hour period. There are 2.5G and 5G preparations, containing 25mg and 50mg respectively. Androgel has been reported in clinical trials to be well tolerated and there have been no problems of sensitivity to sunlight exposure.

Table 1 summarizes the testosterone preparations available in the United States at the time of writing.

Table 1. Currently Available Testosterone Preparations

Oral – Methyl testosterone (Android)	10-50 mg every day
Fluoxymesterone (Halotestin)	5–20 mg every day
Buccal - Methyltestosterone (Oreton Methyl)	5-25 mg every day
Subcutaneous Pellets - long-acting (Testopel)	150-450 mg every 3 months
Short-acting intramuscular (Histerone, Tesamone,Testandro)	10-25 mg 2-3 times a week
Long-acting intramuscular Enanthate or Cypionate	150-200 mg every 2-4 weeks
Topical Non-scrotal patch (Androderm)	2-2.5 mg patch every 24 hrs
Scrotal patch (Testoderm)	4-6 mg patch every 22-24 hrs
Gel (Androgel)	2.5-5g daily

When should Testosterone be given?

Testosterone should be given to older men who are low in testosterone. You may ask, "How low is low?" Different laboratories report different ranges for normality. Commonly, 250- 300 ng/dl is the lower limit for total testosterone. However, discretion and clinical judgment have to be exercised, as a low testosterone level may not produce symptoms of andropause in some men. On the other hand, some men with a low normal level of say 400ng/dl may have andropausal symptoms and it is very justifiable to replace them with testosterone.

It is known that aging causes increased binding of testosterone to a protein called sex hormone binding globulin (SHBG). As a result, free testosterone is lowered in aging. Free testosterone is about 10% of that of total testosterone. Some doctors have the opinion that it is more important to consider the levels of free testosterone, and ignore those of total testosterone, when deciding when to replace with androgens. I personally have not found the free testosterone level to be very useful. First of all, it is a more expensive test. Secondly, I have found some older patients to have low total testosterone and completely normal or even high free testosterone levels. I cannot explain this, but believe that the SHBG binding story in aging may be too simplistic.

When considering hormone replacement therapy in androgen deficient elderly men, one must always consider possible risks versus benefits. Testosterone may potentially stimulate prostate carcinoma or benign prostatic hypertrophy. Hence before starting androgens, your physician should check your prostate and measure the PSA level to ensure you do not have an underlying cancer of the prostate. Because of the potential effects of testosterone on hemoglobin and hematocrit levels, a blood count should also be taken prior to treatment and monitored during replacement therapy. The FSH and LH levels may be measured to confirm that your pituitary is functioning normally and responding appropriately to the low testosterone level. A prolactin level is sometimes measured to exclude a rare pituitary tumor. If at all possible, these tests should be done in the early morning because of diurnal variation of the hormones.

The future of Testosterone

Two decades ago, estrogen replacement therapy was not well established. We faced issues about side effects such as breast and uterine cancer. Further refinements led to combination regimens of estrogens with progestogens. Today, we know that hormonal therapy in women is useful to delay osteoporosis, heart disease and even dementia. At this point in time, testosterone replacement is unfortunately not yet considered routine for the elderly male, but the potential is tremendous. Further research is needed before recommending it routinely for our elderly male patients. At present, a "case by case" approach should be taken, and careful discussion with the physician about the risks and benefits is imperative. Paradoxically, DHEA, which is converted to testosterone in the body, is readily available for purchase over the counter and many patients are taking this as a "health food" without medical supervision. Your doctor should play an important role in educating you about hormone replacement and come up with an appropriate treatment plan. Please consult your doctor before you embark on any testosterone replacement. This is not a treatment that should be unsupervised, as your doctor should be monitoring your blood count and prostate every 2-3 months.

Chapter 8:
Growth Hormone in Old Age

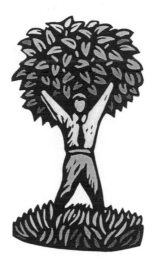

What is Growth Hormone?

As the name suggests, this hormone is involved with the
growing process and in children, growing tall will not be
possible without this hormone. Growth hormone is produced
in the front part of a structure in the brain called the anterior
pituitary gland. Several other hormones are produced in the
anterior pituitary gland including thyroid stimulating
hormone, prolactin, follicular stimulating (FSH) and
luteinizing hormone (LH). The back part of the pituitary or
the posterior pituitary produces two hormones, antidiuretic

hormone (ADH) and oxytonin. Thus in diseases of the pituitary that lead to hypopituitarism (low functioning pituitary gland) several hormones can be affected.

Besides affecting body stature, growth hormone fine-tunes body composition and adjusts the muscle to fat ratio, just like testosterone as described in chapter 2. Growth hormone also modifies blood sugar and body lipids and seems to have a regulatory action on the cardiovascular system. Another function of this hormone is to alter bone mineral density and strengthen bone, similar to testosterone and estrogen. Some investigators have even found that growth hormone influences mental function.

In normal people, sleep and exercise are two major stimuli for secretion of growth hormone and there is evidence to indicate that the growth hormone response to exercise is essential for developing and maintaining physical fitness.

What happens to Growth Hormone with Aging?

A gradual and progressive fall in spontaneous growth hormone secretion occurs with increasing age and is reflected in a parallel fall in insulin- like growth factor (IGF)-I. However, the measurement of IGF-I may not be adequate in determining growth hormone status in the older male, and I will discuss more of this later.

Growth hormone begins to decline gradually approximately between the ages of 25-30 years. Thus it is one of the hormones that start their decline early. Perhaps, it is because once you stop growing taller, the role of growth hormone may not be that important and the body tells it to shut off. However, this shutting off can lead to dire consequences. By the age of 40 years, our growth hormone production is down to 50% of our youthful levels. By the age of 55, it sinks to 20%, so imagine how very low it gets when you are 80! The timing of the Andropause is also related to the fall of growth hormone. With rock-bottom testosterone and growth hormone, life can be tedious and definitely without pep! Part of the reason we sometimes don't realize these hormones are missing in our bodies is because the decline creeps up so very slowly upon us, and we generally attribute how we feel to mere "aging" or getting old.

Some doctors have coined the term "somatopause" to describe the clinical condition associated with declines of growth hormone. Although I acknowledge that this event truly occurs, I do not prefer this terminology as this condition affects both males and females and many of the clinical symptomatology overlaps with the Menopause and Andropause. The Andropause is a time of decline of multiple hormones, and androgens like testosterone are not the only culprits, another is growth hormone.

Can Growth Hormone deficiency cause symptoms?

Certainly. The reason we know this for a fact is because many symptoms disappear on replacement with growth hormone, not unlike replacement with testosterone or estrogen. In children with hypopituitarism, replacement with growth hormone often restores height. In older individuals the growth plates (epiphyses) have fused and further growth is no longer possible, so the symptoms and signs of growth hormone deficiency are more complicated:

a) The lean body mass or muscle is reduced, as muscle building is regulated in part by growth hormone. As a result, overall strength and exercise performance are decreased.

b) Body fat is increased. As muscle disappears, there is a corresponding accumulation of fat.

c) The metabolic rate is lowered, which unfortunately results in yet further accumulation of fat, and sometimes elevation of blood pressure and cholesterol.

d) The bad cholesterol (LDL) is increased and the good cholesterol (HDL) is decreased.

e) There is loss of skin tone, which may result in premature wrinkles. The skin may also become dry and itchy.

f) There is loss of bone mass, leading to osteoporosis

g) Other symptoms associated with growth hormone deficiency include reduced libido, poor general health, memory loss, hair loss and graying.

You may recollect that the lack of testosterone also causes many of these signs and symptoms. Thus in the Andropause, when there is a marked decline in both testosterone and growth hormone, many regulatory processes go amiss. The flip side of this is that there is great potential of reversing some of the effects of aging with hormonal replacement. Not all doctors will agree to hormone replacement for the elderly individual. Some view aging as a "natural process", and that death, like taxes, is inevitable. There is also the potential of abuse as hormone replacement is not without risk, although some would sacrifice everything for the "Elixir of Youth".

What are the other causes of Growth Hormone deficiency?

Aging per se is the commonest cause of natural growth hormone deficiency. However, in younger individuals, a pathological cause for growth hormone deficiency should be carefully sought for. In a study of 172 adults with hypopituitarism, a pituitary tumor was present in 76% of cases. A tumor outside the pituitary called craniopharyngioma accounted for another 13%. Sarcoidosis was the cause in 1%, and Sheehan's syndrome another 1%. The cause was unknown in 8%. Sheehan's syndrome results from excessive bleeding during childbirth, whereas sarcoidosis is an immunological disorder. Hence, although tumors are rare, they should be excluded before one embarks on hormonal replacement.

Diseases of the pituitary gland result in deficiency of growth hormone more often than the other hormones like corticotrophin (ACTH) and thyrotropin (TSH). Some patients with hypopituitarism have done extremely well and have reached a ripe old age because they received regular hormone replacement and did not have to rely on their own inadequate production of growth hormone.

Diagnosing Growth Hormone deficiency

This, I think, presents a bit of a challenge. Not many doctors test their elderly patients for this hormone despite them complaining of the symptoms of growth hormone deficiency. There may be several reasons and I will try to explain them.

a) The cost of a test for Somatomedin C (a growth hormone) is about $85. Add to this a complete blood count, basic chemistry panel, thyroid, PSA and testosterone levels, and the bill suddenly becomes $350! This is apart from the medical consultation and the treatment costs. Those other tests I mentioned are essential for a complete evaluation, especially if one is to contemplate hormonal replacement. Insurance companies and Medicare may not reimburse for these tests unless they are deemed "medically necessary". Whether aging should be regarded as a "disease" or a "natural process" is highly debatable, and there are valid arguments from both sides.

c) There is no general agreement among doctors as to which test is best. It is like the story of free testosterone and total testosterone. The purist insists that the diagnosis can only be made when there is "below normal serum responses to two provocative stimuli". Simply measuring serum IGF-I or basal growth hormone may not be enough. The basis of this purist view is from a study of 200 adults with proven growth hormone deficiency, where up to 51% patients actually had a serum IGF-I concentration in the normal range. For this reason, the purist would argue for ***provocative tests.*** These tests should be performed in the morning after an overnight fast, and an important caveat is that obesity may produce abnormal provocative tests in the absence of growth hormone deficiency. The provocation can be achieved by several means, including insulin-induced hypoglycemia, intravenous arginine infusion, L-DOPA, clonidine and glucagon. These provocative tests are complicated and most doctors are not familiar with these tests. The shortcut method of diagnosis, namely by doing a single measurement of growth hormone and the analogues may produce inaccurate results. My sense is that if the symptoms are very suggestive of deficiency and a basal level of growth hormone confirms very low levels, a provocative test may be unnecessary.

d) A month's worth of growth hormone may cost from $1000-$3000, and not many individuals can afford this. It is easy to justify replacement with growth hormone if, for instance, a patient suffers from hypopituitarism secondary to a tumor. Most insurance plans will not deny this prescription benefit. However, if an older individual is low on growth hormone because of the aging process and not because of a pituitary tumor, it is harder to justify the prescription benefit, and insurance company do not see this as a medical necessity. As such, many people who seek the hormone turn to private anti-aging clinics, which charge a fee for their services. Some of them are shams and many patients get short-changed, sometimes even getting products other than growth hormone. Others have gone across the border to Mexico and Canada to purchase this elixir of youth.

The effects of Growth Hormone replacement in Men over 60 years

In all my years of clinical practice, I have not found one drug that is perfectly safe 100% of the time. Even over the counter drugs like Tylenol and vitamins may do harm if taken in excessive amounts or not in the recommended way. Growth Hormone is a very powerful drug and potentially has some serious side effects.

The landmark study on the effects of human growth hormone in men over 60 years was published in the July 5, 1990 issue of the New England Journal of Medicine. Dr. Rudman and his colleagues conducted the study at the Medical College of Wisconsin in Milwaukee. They believed that the declining activity of growth hormone with advancing age led to the loss of body mass and an increase in fat. This study in a sense was very similar to the studies on testosterone of the 1940's, which were published in the Journal of the American Medical Association.

Dr. Rudman and colleagues studied 21 men aged between 61 to 81 years old, with plasma IGF-I levels less than 350 U/L. One group of 12 men received 0.03mg per kilogram body weight of the biosynthetic human growth hormone, given subcutaneously three times a week. The control group of 9 men received no treatment. Every month for 6 months, both groups had their plasma IGF-I, lean body mass, bone density fat and skin thickness measured.

In the group treated with growth hormone, the average plasma IGF-I level rose to the youthful range of between 400- 1500 IU/L. The untreated group had an average IGF-I level remaining low at less than 350IU/L. In addition, the treated group had an 8.8% increase in lean body mass and a 14.4 per cent decrease in adipose mass. Moreover a 1.6% bone density increase was noticed in the lumbar spine in the treated group, and skin thickness was increased by 7.1%.

Replacement with Growth Hormone in the Andropause

Do the results of Dr. Rudman's study suggest that all men in the Andropause receive growth hormone? Is it right to deny or delay aging? Unlike estrogen therapy, growth hormone replacement has not caught on as routine hormonal replacement.

The authors of the study themselves wrote a letter in the May issue of the Journal of the American Geriatrics Society saying that there were many unanswered questions concerning the treatment of low growth hormone levels in elderly men. In a paper published in the October 1993 issue of Clinical Endocrinology, the same group issued warnings that after elderly men received growth hormone continuously, many patients developed carpal tunnel syndrome and gynaecomastia. In other words, many older males started getting numbness in the hands and breast enlargement. By their estimate, approximately one in four developed carpal tunnel syndrome and one in ten developed breasts. A few others developed high blood sugar (diabetes).

At this point, you may want to ask yourself if you should really be on growth hormone or not. I have heard testimonies of patients who swear that they have never felt better or looked more youthful than after receiving growth hormone. At present this treatment is largely reserved for the few who can afford the huge cost. Medicare and most insurance companies do not pay for this medication which is not FDA approved at the moment. The side effects are there but so are the potential benefits. Before you even consider putting yourself on growth hormone, ask yourself these questions:

1. Are the risks worth the potential gains?
2. Am I willing to pay for the medication?

3. Am I not willing to accept aging, and are there other ways of aging graciously?
4. Am I comfortable injecting myself, and being supervised closely by my doctor?

There are many other preparations of "growth hormone" that are available. Some are worthless imitations of the real thing, which has to be bioengineered through elaborate biotechnological processes. There are some oral medications called secretogues that claim to improve natural growth hormone production. In the horizon are some very new novel drugs, thanks again to cutting-edge biotechnology. These drugs work on the growth hormone receptor and help the body produce the natural growth hormone. Perhaps this might be the answer, to coax the body to continue producing growth hormone instead of shutting down, which occurs in the Andropause. It will be interesting to see if "naturally produced hormone" would be safer and not have the side effects of the synthetic growth hormone. A true elixir of youth may be found, pending clinical trials on humans.

Side effects and monitoring of Growth Hormone replacement

We talked briefly about the side effects of growth hormone above. A condition called Acromegaly or adult gigantism occurs because there is a tumor of the pituitary gland. This tumor leads to an excess of growth hormone and causes the body to grow abnormally. The jaw protrudes and the face becomes big and distorted. The hands also become very large and skin over the hands slowly become thick and coarse. This thickening of the tissues in the hands causes a nerve called the median nerve to be trapped, resulting in the carpal tunnel syndrome. Typically the outer 3½ finger portions of the hand are affected with numbness and tingling. Acromegalics also develop high blood pressure, diabetes and heart disease. Hence they often do not live the normal life span and often die of heart failure.

Of course growth hormone should not be replaced to the levels that will turn you into an acromegalic! Rather, it should be restored only to levels of your youth so that you do not suffer from side effects. Therefore if you are on growth hormone, your doctor should monitor your blood pressure, blood sugar and heart carefully. Your bone mass, body weight and skin fat should be assessed before and during treatment. Your growth hormone profile, such as IGF-I level, should be measured regularly so that adequate amounts of growth hormone are given, and not excessive.

Possible benefits in Post-Polio Syndrome

Polio or poliomyelitis is a viral disease that no longer strikes in epidemic proportions in developed countries with an active vaccination program. However, in less developed countries cases still erupt. This disease is a very crippling disease affecting the anterior horn cells of the spinal cord, leading to permanent muscle weakness.

In the United States vaccination against polio was not widely available until the 1950-60's. Hence there are many survivors of polio living today, many of which walk with a limp or need crutches, braces or even a wheel chair. In post-polio syndrome there is often weakness in the muscles, muscle twitching and easy fatigue.

Research has shown that survivors of polio have lower levels of IGF-I than compared with their similar-aged cohorts. There may be a potential role of growth hormone in the post-polio syndrome, in that replacement with growth hormone may possibly alleviate some of the distressing symptoms. A study showed no consistent benefits, but some individuals did find relief, perhaps demonstrating that this drug holds some promise for sufferers.

Chapter 9:
Diet & Supplements for the Andropause

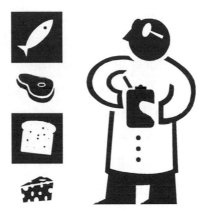

Eat healthy

Eating healthy is the key to a fit life. As a Geriatrician, I see a lot of self-induced diseases in older people as a result of poor dietary habits. For example, obesity aggravates arthritis and heart disease, iron deficiency causes anemia and vitamin B12 deficiency causes neurological problems.

It honestly is very simple. Remember the basic food groups: protein, carbohydrate and fat. Body muscle is made up of protein, and unfortunately many andropausal men do not consume enough protein to replace the muscle mass that is being lost as part of the aging process. Common reasons include the gradual loss of dental strength as well as the blunting of taste buds that is inevitable with aging, and it becomes harder and harder to devour that 8 oz. steak which seemed so small when we were in our twenties! Convenient alternatives are protein supplements in the form of pills and drinks, such as Ensure and Boost, but be careful not to overload your kidneys with too much protein especially if you have kidney failure. If you feel you are not consuming enough protein, you should consult a physician or a dietitian.

Carbohydrate is easy fuel and readily burns up and satisfies the appetite. But if you consume too much carbohydrate, the excess that is not burnt up as fuel gets stored as fat. Diets high in sugar and refined carbohydrates like donuts, cereal, cakes and cookies increase your body's production of insulin. When insulin levels in the body are high, the food you eat gets readily converted into body fat, in the form of triglycerides. A high triglyceride level is one of the greatest risk factors for heart disease, so beware! Ironically, high carbohydrate meals tend to leave you less satisfied than those that contain adequate protein and fat, so you tend to eat more but get hungrier sooner. A typical example is gorging yourself with pasta at lunch, and then surprisingly getting so hungry in the mid-afternoon that you run to the vending machine for another "carbohydrate-fix". Somehow all that pasta you ate could not get you to stay full until dinnertime. So the typical high-carbohydrate, low-protein and low-fat meal leaves you eating more but getting hungrier sooner.

So, in a poor diet, the worst offenders are sugar, white flour and other refined carbohydrate-based products. By getting off the insulin-generating roller coaster of the low-fat diet and cutting down on carbohydrate consumption, there will be wonderful results:

1. You will start to burn fat for energy. If carbohydrates are the body's primary energy source, you will rarely utilize the secondary energy source, your own body fat. But if you restrict carbohydrate consumption, you will get the body fat to burn, and successfully lose weight.

2. You won't feel hungry in between meals. A big battle that many people struggle with is the constant obsession with food, for example already thinking about dinner when still eating lunch. Much of this is caused by blood sugar fluctuations aggravated by excessive carbohydrate consumption, especially of refined carbohydrates. By cutting down on carbohydrates, you'll maintain a more constant blood sugar level throughout the day, with no more between-meal hunger pains or brain drains.

3. Your overall health will improve and you'll feel better. Many of the toxins in your body are stored in the fat cells. By getting your body to burn stored fat, you activate a self-cleansing process. As a result many common ailments such as fatigue, irritability, depression, headaches, and even joint and muscular pain could well be alleviated. Furthermore, you could see a significant improvement in your cholesterol and blood pressure levels, leading to better health and general well being.

Fat is essential for the body, but in excess, it clogs up your arteries and distorts your physique. Many of you may not realize this, but the male hormones are derived from cholesterol, so don't deprive yourself completely of all cholesterol either, as life will be no fun. There may be some truth that foods such as lobster tails, oysters and caviar have aphrodisiac functions, because after all, they are full of cholesterol! Please keep a balance though, as eating too much oysters can clog up your arteries including the penile ones, which will result in vascular impotence.

Remember that a wealth of antioxidants is found in fresh fruits and vegetables, and that a high fiber diet will also help in preventing dementia, cancer and heart disease. Lifestyle modification is necessary in the Andropause. If you need to eat out often, plan where to do so in advance, rather than resorting to a fast-food meal on impulse. Have a diary of the meals for the week ahead and prepare in advance so that you keep the right balance. Take time to discuss this with your spouse or partner if she is doing the shopping and cooking so that you both make a habit of eating healthy.

Should I take supplements in the Andropause?

There are many different types of supplements out there, all available without a prescription, so you don't even need to see your doctor for them. Research has shown that 40-60% of men take some kind of dietary supplement, which makes this an undeniably important topic. Let me briefly describe a few supplements that may have an impact on the Andropause.

DHEA

This is the abbreviation for dihydroepiandrosterone. This substance is very closely related chemically to testosterone and actually breaks down in the body to become testosterone. DHEA is involved in several functions, including immune system support, tissue maintenance and repair as well as mental support. Just like testosterone, DHEA peaks at the time of puberty and early adulthood, and then declines with aging. DHEA is manufactured in the body by the adrenals glands and cannot be found in any food substance. Most of the commercial DHEA is made synthetically in the laboratory from Mexican wild yams. Fresh yams per se don't have the hormone so it will be futile going to the supermarket and buying a whole bagful of yams in an attempt to boost your libido!

There have been speculations that DHEA may help with erectile dysfunction. The Massachusetts Male Aging Study found an inverse relationship of DHEA levels and the incidence of erectile dysfunction. In other words, there was a higher rate of erectile dysfunction in men with lower DHEA levels. Anther study from Austria published in Urology also supported this notion, and anecdotally, some of my patients have told me that their sexuality improved with DHEA.

However, there have not been really good trials to support that DHEA improves erectile dysfunction, although it may well do so. Low DHEA levels may also be a risk factor for developing Alzheimer's disease as demonstrated in a study performed in Germany (Biology Psychiatry Jan 2000), and hence DHEA may improve memory for some patients.

DHEA should never be consumed if you have a prostate disorder or cancer. This supplement also has other side effects, such as acne, unwanted hair growth in women, breast enlargement in men, mood swings and lethargy.

If you decide to buy this medicine off the shelf, I would strongly suggest you see your physician to be checked for prostate cancer first before starting this supplement. I have heard of patients developing prostate cancer from consuming DHEA without supervision. In my study on the perceptions of the Andropause, I found that most men did not consider that it was illegal to attain a hormone like DHEA over the counter without a prescription. Most men feel that they don't really need medical supervision to consume hormones but they do! There are dangerous risks when taking this supplement without supervision.

Melatonin

This is a hormone secreted by the pineal gland, a pea-sized organ in the brain. This hormone controls many functions including your precious sleep, and also has antioxidant properties that protect your immune system. The suggested dose is 0.1 to 0.3 mg, but there is no agreed dosage as to what is optimal for antioxidation. By and large, melatonin is very safe but it may cause drowsiness in some individuals. In other instances, it may aggravate depressive symptoms, particularly in some psychiatric patients.

In the andropausal years, your sleep habits tend to get disrupted and this hormone may help restore some regularity. If you are planning a long trip on a plane over several time zones, it may be an antidote to jet lag. Moreover in selected patients, it may improve depression and even memory. There are claims that melatonin may combat cancer but so far, there has been no concrete scientific proof of this.

Gingko Biloba

This is an extract from a tree that has existed for several thousands of years. This tree grows in many parts of the United States and may even be found in your backyard or neighborhood park. Researchers have found that the extract from the gingko leaf interferes with the action of platelet activating factor (PAF), a compound the body produces. Inhibiting PAF may retard some of the aging processes of the Andropause.

Many people take Gingko to combat memory loss. A study published in the December 1992 issue of Lancet suggested that Gingko could reverse memory loss in

Alzheimer's disease. In normal people, Gingko can improve brain function by improving blood circulation in the brain. This herb is also an antioxidant and can help retard heart disease and cancer.

Some researchers have found that Gingko has some antidepressant effects and can improve moods. This herb is believed to reverse depression by normalizing levels of neurotransmitters. A recent study form San Francisco has demonstrated that Gingko can partially retard and counteract the sexual dysfunction caused by antidepressants. To be specific, it was found that the erectile dysfunction and loss of libido caused by Prozac could be corrected by Gingko. This may be important information for andropausal men who are on antidepressants.

In addition, some of my non-depressed patients have claimed that Gingko has helped them with erectile dysfunction. This may be because Gingko acts by improving circulation to the penis, not unlike Viagra. I do recommend my andropausal patients to be on Gingko because by and large, this is a safe drug especially at recommended dosages. However, if you take more than 40mg/day, you are at risk of headaches, abdominal upset and diarrhea. Also, be especially cautious if you have a clotting disorder or are on anticoagulant medication, like aspirin or coumadin, as excessive bleeding may be caused when taken in conjunction with Gingko. As always, consult your physician before you decide to be on any supplements.

Saw Palmetto

Saw Palmetto comes from a small palm tree native to Florida and the Gulf Coast. It produces a brownish berry and has been used by Native Americans for centuries to treat urinary symptoms. In the 1960's researchers found that the saw palmetto fruit contained fatty acids that help counteract prostate enlargement.

Many men take Saw Palmetto during the Andropause because they are starting to have problems with their prostate. The prostate is a gland situated just above the bladder and when it enlarges, it causes blockage to the flow of urine, a clinical situation called prostatism. There have been many studies supporting the efficacy of Saw Palmetto, but most of these trials were performed in Europe. In general Europeans tend to be more skeptical of conventional medicine and are more receptive to herbal medications than Americans. Two studies, one done in France and another in Germany, compared Saw Palmetto to Proscar (a conventional medicine for prostatism), and both showed that the effectiveness of Saw Palmetto was close to that of Proscar in reducing urinary obstructive symptoms. This supplement is essentially safe in standard dosages (160mg) but may cause abdominal upset. Again, if you are taking this to treat yourself of urinary symptoms during the Andropause, consult your physician first, as cancer of the prostate can cause urinary obstruction in rare instances and must be excluded.

St. John's Wort

Depression is a problem many andropausal men struggle with. St. John's wort has been shown to help people suffering from various stages of depression. A German study demonstrated that St. John's wort was only slightly less effective than the antidepressant drug imipramine. Conversely, an Austrian study showed that St. John's wort was better than placebo in reversing depression. One advantage of St. John's wort is the low incidence of side effects, as currently known. Tricyclic antidepressants are not be suitable for heart patients, and SSRI antidepressants may cause side effects including loss of appetite.

The dose that was used in previous research was 300mg up to three times a day. The supplement may not be effective until after 4 weeks of consumption, not unlike prescription antidepressants. I know of several physicians who are treating their own depression with St. John's wort rather than with prescription antidepressants. I suspect many people, including physicians, still feel the stigma of seeing a psychiatrist and getting a prescription antidepressant, so they prefer to manage the problem themselves and purchase an over-the-counter supplement which is by and large safe.

St. John's wort has been in use for more than 2000 years. The leaves and flowers of St. John's wort contain special glands that release red oil. Early Christians named it after John the Baptist because the plant released its blood-red oil during the anniversary of the Saint's beheading. Over the centuries, St. John's wort has been used to treat wounds, and also has had a part in protecting against witches spells.

If you take St. John's wort and have heart disease, be careful as it may interact with digoxin, a medication used to treat congestive heart failure. Some patients have reported abdominal pains, allergic reactions, fatigue and restlessness as side effects. If you are taking this supplement in the Andropause or are suffering from depression, please discuss this with your physician.

Garlic

Garlic is used in many cultures in everyday cooking. From the Mediterranean to the Far East, this plant has been used for centuries. The Egyptians were probably the highest consumers of garlic recorded in history. In Numbers 11:5 of the Old Testament, it is recorded: "We remember the fish we had eaten in Egypt, and also the cucumbers, melons, leeks, onions and garlic". Greeks were also large consumers, and athletes ate it before races.

Garlic contains allin, which by itself is an inactive ingredient. However, when allin comes in contact with the enzyme allinase, it is converted to allicin, which is the source of the healing power of garlic. Garlic is believed to have several functions, including lowering cholesterol levels, improving digestion and protecting from infections, heart attacks, strokes and possibly cancer.

161

Blood pressure and cholesterol become major issues in the fifties and sixties, coinciding with the timing of the Andropause. Hence many andropausal men suffer from heart disease, for whom this could be a worthwhile supplement. Usually100mg capsules taken three times daily are sufficient and probably less offensive than fresh garlic, but fresh garlic is obviously much cheaper, although you risk losing your partner and your friends!

Vitamin E

Vitamin E is also known as tocopherol, which in Greek, translates to "to reproduce". Unfortunately, the reproductive potential of this supplement has only been verified in laboratory rats, and it has not restored fertility in post-andropausal men. Vitamin E is a well-known antioxidant, and the different grades of antioxidant capacities of Vitamin E are based on the classifications - alpha tocopherols are better at antioxidizing than beta and so on. According to the free radical theory, free oxygen radicals damage cells in the body and antioxidants may retard this, thereby slowing the processes of aging. Vitamin E is one of the four fat-soluble vitamins and is found in dark green vegetables, eggs, fish, nuts, meats, soya and wheat based products. The recommended daily allowance is 8-10mg per day and for most people on a well-balanced diet, there is no need for Vitamin E supplementation. However, for older individuals whose diets are less than adequate or when dental problems limit adequate food intake, supplementation is advised.

Vitamin E may have several functions including the production of red blood cells, antioxidant and anti-aging properties, and anticoagulant or blood thinning properties. Hence you have to be careful if you are already on anticoagulants like warfarin, as Vitamin E may interact and cause prolonged bleeding. A high intake of Vitamin E and A can also interfere with B-carotene absorption.

If you are taking Vitamin E, it will be prudent to also take Vitamin C and selenium, which may enhance the antioxidant function of Vitamin E. Do not take Vitamin E with mineral oils as the latter will decrease absorption of the former. If iron is taken simultaneously, the Vitamin E may be oxidized and thus inactivated, so do not consume both these supplements in the same gulp.

Aspirin

This wonder drug has been around for a long time, primarily for pain relief. It was not until a clinical trial, done initially in the United Kingdom, but repeated in the United States, during which doctors put themselves on this drug, that made the world realize its important potential of saving lives. Today, aspirin is used to prevent heart attacks, blood clots and even strokes. This is achieved by inhibiting a prostaglandin, thus preventing blood vessels from closing or narrowing. In the andropausal years, many men are at risk of suffering heart attacks and strokes, chiefly because of longstanding high blood pressure and cholesterol problems, although hormones may be partly responsible. Often a daily pediatric dose (81mg) of aspirin is enough and the enteric-coated formulation taken after food is safer to prevent gastrointestinal bleeding. In fact aspirin is notorious for causing dangerous bleeding especially if you already have stomach problems like an ulcer, so consult your physician before you start yourself on aspirin.

Chapter 10:

Secrets beyond Andropause: Actually it is no Mystery !

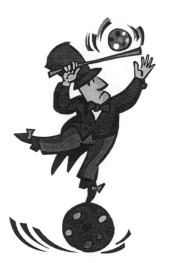

Stress in the Andropause

The female readers of this book will probably agree with me for saying that men are very complex and fragile beings. Conversely I am sure men make the same remark about women. In any event as the older male ages and undergoes the Andropause, he has to grapple with profound changes and issues, as elaborated in earlier chapters. All changes bring about stress, and if stress is not managed well, it can be very disabling and even lead to depression.

I firmly believe there should be no mystery to progressing gracefully through this critical phase of a man's life, so to help combat the stress and challenges of the Andropause, I am offering the following six simple strategies.

Six Simple Strategies to combat Stress in the Andropause

1. Love and Reward yourself
2. Take Control and Organize yourself
3. Exercise yourself
4. Relax and Rest yourself
5. Feed yourself
6. Enjoy the Andropause

---

1. Love and Reward yourself

Research has shown that people who love themselves generally do better. Perhaps they produce more brain transmitters such as serotonin, noradrenalin and dopamine, which are the body's natural "uppers". When a man undergoes changes during the andropausal years, he has to learn to accept and love his evolving self. Moreover, as you learn to love yourself, learn to love others too. Be especially considerate to your spouse or partner as she is aging in parallel, and likely to be suffering from multifold changes herself. Try to spend as much time as possible with children and grandchildren, if you have any. Their innocence and playful nature will make you feel younger and more invigorated!

Along with loving yourself, learn to reward yourself. The Andropause should be a time for celebration for now is the time to reward all the previous years of hard work. At this point in life, many older males have fewer problems with finances, particularly if they worked and saved for a lifetime. If you have always wanted help for a particular task, or travel to a certain place, or do a special activity, then go ahead and do it! You now have the disposable income you never had before, and you won't be able to take any of it with you to the Afterlife. Remember how, in earlier years, you had to struggle with mortgage payments? Well now is the time to enjoy your previous thrift, and buy that cottage, boat or recreational vehicle that you always yearned for. However, please do everything in balance, for a new acquisition can itself lead to more stress, as it too leads to changes in your lifestyle. Don't forget that any *change* can bring on stress.

As you give yourself treats, keep in mind to treat others too. Much joy can come from giving because as you give, you can attain deep satisfaction and this ultimately is a form of rewarding yourself. Give yourself to your spouse, friends and family, and where feasible, extend that to the community you live in and the church in your neighborhood. Reward yourself with your own personal dreams, like that cottage by the lake and that boat. But reward others too, as by doing so you double the pleasure.

2. Take Control and Organize yourself

A multitude of changes occur during the Andropause, but most can be resolved provided you take charge and exert control. For example, it may be that you have to be firm and stay away from alcohol. The andropausal years may bring about so much stress that many resort to alcoholism. Being retired, having more free time and not knowing what to do, is a risk for alcoholism, so beware! Often alcohol is exchanged for a good diet, thereby causing weakness because of poor nutrition. Moreover, it can worsen your memory, and may even result in a condition called alcohol dementia. It is true that in moderate amounts of up to 2 drinks a day, alcohol can help with sex drive and protect the heart, but please stay away from excessive consumption.

If you have an alcohol problem, see your doctor as soon as possible. Studies have shown that older men are at least as likely to benefit from treatment than younger men. The outcomes are more favorable in people with a shorter history of drinking, that is, they took up drinking later in life. Unfortunately the usefulness of drugs for treating alcoholism has not been very consistent. In particular, Antabuse should be avoided as it can affect the heart of the older patient. Having said that, there recently have been reports of success with naltrexone (ReVia) in reversing alcoholism in some older individuals.

Excessive smoking is another disastrous pitfall to be firmly avoided, as it hastens your development of Andropausal symptoms by as much as 5 years. If you recall the chapter on erectile dysfunction, we discussed how smoking compromises blood flow to the penis and that vascular causes are the most common of erectile dysfunction. Some of you may have tried to quit smoking but were unsuccessful. It is extremely difficult because nicotine in cigarettes is a highly addictive drug. But don't loose heart because quitting cigarettes is a learning curve for most, and it takes effort, time and total commitment. By and large, most people take 2 - 3 attempts before they finally quit. Some medications can help you to stop smoking by lessening your urge to smoke. Of the ones that are FDA approved, Buproprion (Zyban) requires a prescription, whereas nicotine inhaler, spray, gum and patch are all available over the counter. There are also some alternatives to medications. Several patients of mine have tried acupuncture and report great success. The needles are tiny and may be placed on your ear, so that overall, the procedure is relatively painless and well tolerated.

Apart from taking control in the areas of alcohol and smoking, there are a host of issues where you may need to be proactive. Perhaps you should be consulting your physician to determine if you have a problem with hormones, for which hormonal replacement may be highly appropriate. The onus will be on you to make that first appointment! Perhaps you still work, but are feeling pushed around in the job and the mounting stress is making it less and less enjoyable by the day. Perhaps this is the time to spell out the word "retirement", so that you can now really go smell the roses! You have already worked hard all your life, so now it is the time of the Andropause, to be enjoyed and not suffered!

To combat changes in your life during the andropausal years, try to organize yourself so that you are the one in control. One common major change could be that all of a sudden you are retired and at a loss for day-to-day motivation and mission. Organize your time by planning your day or week ahead. For the technologically inclined, invest in a Palm Pilot™. For those technically challenged a good simple diary will work just as adequately. Anticipating events before they unexpectedly befall you is one way to combat stress. On the other hand, you might be even busier during the andropausal years because you are now trying to catch up with lost time and enjoying yourself as much as you can. This may lead to more stress, as there are more changes to face, such as organizing that fishing trip, or the vacation to the pyramids in Egypt. You should plan even your local trips and mundane errands, so for example, you target the stores the same day you visit the dentist. It is also very important to do your estate planning, wills and also your advance directives while you are still feeling well. This way, by staying organized, you effectively battle with time in your andropausal years!

3. Exercise yourself

Exercise is of paramount importance in the andropausal years. Remember what happens to you as you age - muscle is lost and fat is gained Exercise not only strengthens your muscles, which in turn can result in better overall well-being and sexual functioning, but it also preserves your mobility. Research on older individuals has demonstrated that muscles may get bigger in old age, although they do not grow more. That is good news for those in the andropausal years as falls and debility can be minimized. In addition, as you exercise not only is more serotonin, noradrenalin besides dopamine is produced by the brain, but also endorphin, which is a natural hormone known to combat pain and stress. Hence even the pain of arthritis in the andropausal years may lessen with appropriate exercise!

What kind of exercise is best? I believe there should be a combination of both muscle building with weights and cardiovascular building, such as with walking, running or swimming. Research has shown that for exercise to be effective, it has to be done regularly 3 times a week for 15 minutes each time. If the weather is bad outside, you could drive to an indoor mall and comfortably walk several laps. Chances are, you will find good company there as many other people are walking there too. There are also excellent gymnasiums around where you can engage a personal trainer to tailor an exercise program specifically suitable for you. With aging joints often degenerate and you may suffer from osteoporosis and arthritis. In this case it is best to participate in sports that are NOT weight bearing, the ideal being swimming. Whatever the exercise activity, you should start gently and slowly, and gradually build up to a peak. Your body may give you the signals as to when to quit, so listen to it carefully and don't be over enthusiastic.

4. Relax and Rest yourself

When changes occur around us and we loose control, we justifiably get very uptight. One of the keys to avoid stress is to relax. Try to chill out and let go, because in reality, there are other things in life that are much more important than these trivial events. If you really cannot relax, ask for help and see a counselor or your doctor. There are many techniques for relaxation including closing your eyes and breathing slowly and deeply. Another common technique is to close your eyes and initially clench your fists tightly. Then slowly open your clenched fists and imagine all your worries disappearing. Perhaps you should not take yourself too seriously - learn to relax, be funny and laugh at yourself.

In the andropausal years your sleep pattern may change. You may find yourself napping more frequently and sleeping in short but multiple periods. What is important is not so much the frequency of sleep but the total amount of quality sleep. It is the Rapid Eye Movement (REM) sleep that is most important, as this is when your brain rests. In the andropause, a man experiences increased awakenings at night and decreased sleep efficiency. He may take longer to fall asleep and when he finally does, he has decreased REM sleep. As a result, he will find any opportunity he can get to catch up with sleep and may drop off in front of the television, or reading the newspaper or whilst waiting in the car. A few prescribed drugs can adversely affect the REM sleep, even sleeping pills, which is ironical, so these should be avoided if possible. It is much better to rely on mental

172

techniques like counting sheep, daytime exercise to tire yourself, and avoiding caffeine late at night. In fact all drinks should be avoided late at night because if you have to get up to the bathroom often, this disrupt your sleep.

5. Feed yourself

Encouraging you to feed yourself in the Andropause may seem paradoxical as obesity tends to be a frequent problem. Typically by this time, body fat has accumulated in exchange for muscle mass, but it is precisely for this reason that it is important to adjust your diet correctly in the andropausal years. So what is the ideal body weight? Researchers have put together a body mass index (BMI) and have correlated it with health trends like longevity versus dying. The higher up the BMI scale, the greater chance you face of ill health and dying. Thirty is the magic number for severe obesity, and 27 is the cut off for obesity. To check your own BMI, go to www.heliohealth.com and enter in your weight, height and age - the calculations will be done automatically for you.

How do we loose weight in the Andropause? Knowing your calories is very important. Eating in excess of what your body needs or can burn up will result in the accumulation of fat. The Atkins Diet is a scheme I recommend some of my obese andropausal patients, having tried it myself and successfully lost 30 pounds, which I have since kept off. This diet is a lifetime nutritional philosophy, focusing on the consumption of nutrient-dense unprocessed foods together with vita-nutrient supplementation. The Atkins diet restricts processed and refined carbohydrates, which often make up over 50% of a person's diet, such as high-sugar foods, breads, pasta, cereal, and starchy vegetables. Core vita-nutrient supplementation includes a full-spectrum multi-vitamin and an essential oils-fatty acid formula.

Although increased protein intake will help regenerate lost muscles, unfortunately, andropausal years coincide with the lost of teeth, and chewing meat may be difficult and unenjoyable. See your dentist and have good dentures. As an alternative, take protein replacement in liquid forms such as Ensure or Carnation drinks, as they go a long way in building your body. Consume adequate amounts of vegetables and fruits as they not only help in constipation, which can be another unwelcomed stressor, but they also provide a rich source of vitamins and antioxidants.

6. Enjoy the Andropause

Last but not least, ENJOY YOURSELF in the Andropause! This is perhaps the best time in your life as there is now no need to work if you are retired, and no children to worry about as they are all grown up. You may have a retirement fund that has done well in the booming stock market of recent years, and there is now the freedom to travel and do whatever you desire. Although the hormonal changes you are experiencing may be robbing you of some enjoyment, much can be corrected by combating stress, and with a little help from hormone replacement if appropriate.

In reality, there may come a point when we have to accept things just as they are. After all, we are but mortals, and the Andropause is only one of the many chapters in our lives. Depending on your religious belief, this may be a valuable and crucial time of spiritual renewal for you. This chapter may be a journey that is long for some, but short for others, there is no way of predicting. Illness and death may befall us regardless of what we do. Science and medicine often have good answers, but not all the answers and not all the time. Most of us will have to pass through this journey so let us make the best of it. May we make this journey of profound change one also of positive evolvement, and a time of rich blessings for ourselves as well as those around us, as we age graciously through the Andropause!

SELECTED BIBLIOGRAPHY

Many journals, magazines and books were reviewed for this work. The author acknowledges the work of these scientists and opinion leaders. Following are some references that might be useful for your further reading.

Chapter 1

1) Jenkins T. Male menopause: myth or monster? *Vibrant Life* 1995; 11 (6): 12-13

2) Vermeulen A, Rubens R, Verdonck L. Testosterone secretion and metabolism in male senescence. *J Clin Endocrinol Metab* 1972; 34: 730-735

3) Gray A, Feldman HA, McKinlay JB et al. Age, disease, and changing sex hormone levels in middle-aged men: Results of the Massachusetts Male Aging Study. *J Clin Endocrinol Metab* 1991; 73: 1016-1025

4) Bremner WJ, Vitiello MV, Pronz PN. Loss of circadian rhythmicity in blood testosterone levels with aging in normal men. *J Clin Endocrinol Metab* 1983; 56: 1278-1281

5) Tan R. Pathological fracture due to testosterone deficiency in an elderly man. Abstract from the annual scientific meeting of the American Geriatrics Society 1997

6) Vermeulen A. The Male Climacterium. *Annals of Medicine* 1993; 25: 531- 534

7) Vermeulen A, Rubens R, Verdonck L. Testosterone secretion and metabolism in male senescence. *J Clin Endocrinol Metab* 1972; 34: 730-5

8) Burns Cox, Gingell C. The Andropause: fact or fiction? *Postgrad Med J* 1997; (863): 553- 6

9) Matsumoto AM, Hormonal therapy of male hypogonadism. *Endocrinol Metab Clin North Am* 1994; 33(4):857- 75.

10) Heller CG, Myers G. The male climacteric , its symptomatology, diagnosis and treatment. *JAMA* 1944; 126(8): 472- 477

11) La Haye In*: Understanding the Male Temperament*, New Jersey, Power Books, 1977.

Chapter 2

1) Kenney RA. In: Physiology of Aging, 2nd ed. Chicago: Year Book Publishers Inc, 1989

2) Rubinow DR, Schmidt PJ. Androgens, Brain and Behavior. *Am J Psychiatry* 1996; 153(8): 974-84

3) West JB. In: Physiological basis of medical practice, 12th ed. Baltimore: Willliams & Wilkins, 1991: 820-832

4) Tenover JS. Effects of testosterone supplementation in the aging male. *J Clin Endocrinol Metab* 1992; 75: 1092

5) Wilson WD, Roehrborn C. Long term consequences of castration in men: Lessons from the Skoptzy and the Eunuchs of the Chinese and Ottoman Courts. *J Clin Endocrinol & Metab* 1999; 84(12): 4324- 4331

6) Brown Sequard. The effects on man by subcutaneous injections of a liquid obtained from the testicles of animals. *The Lancet* 1889; July 20: 105-107

Chapter 3

1) Cowley RA. Lifestyle/My month on DHEA. *Newsweek* September 16, 1996.

2) Nedstrand E, Pertl J, Hammar M. Climacteric symptoms in a postmenopausal Czech population. *Mauritas* 1996; 23 (1): 85-9.

3) Alvardo ZG, Rivera Damm R, Ruiz MR et al. Factors possibly associated with the age at onset of menopause. Multicenter study. *Ginecol Obstet Mex* 1995; 63: 432- 8.

4) Cramer DW, Harlow BL, Xu H et al. Cross sectional and case controlled analyses of the association between smoking and early menopause. *Maturitas* 1995: 22(2): 79- 87.

5) Morales A, Heaton JP, Carson CC. Andropause: A misnomer for a true clinical entity *J Clin Endocrinol & Metab* 2000; 163: 705-712.

6) Tan RS, Philip P: Perceptions of, and risk factors for the Andropause. *Archives of Andrology* 1999, 43(2): 97-103.

Chapter 4

1) Janowsky JS, Oviatt SK, Orwoll ES. Testosterone influences spatial cognition in older men. *Behav- Neurosci* 1994; 108 (2): 325- 332

2) Rocca WA et al. Epidemiology of clinically diagnosed Alzheimer's Disease. *Ann Neural* 1986; 19: 415.

3) Snowdon DA, Greiner LH, Mortimer JA et al. Brain infarction and the clinical expression of Alzheimer's disease. The Nun Study. *Journal American Medical Association* 1997, 277(10): 277: 813-7.

4) Simpkins JW, Green PS, Gridley KE et al. Role of estrogen replacement therapy in memory enhancement and the prevention of neuronal loss associated with Alzheimer's disease. *American Journal of Medicine* 1997; 103(3A): 19S-25S.

5) Henderson VW, Paganini- Hill A, Emanuel CK et al. Estrogen replacement therapy in older women. Comparisons between Alzheimer's disease and nondemented control subjects. *Arch Neurol* 1994; 51 (9): 896- 900.

6) Mortel KF, Meyer JS. Lack of postmenopausal estrogen replacement therapy and the risk of dementia. *J Neuropsychiatry Clin Neurosci* 1995; 7 (3): 334- 7.

7) Kawas C, Resnick S, Morrsion A et al. A prospective study of estrogen replacement therapy and the risk of developing Alzheimer's disease. The Baltimore Longitudinal Study of Aging. *Neurology* 1997; 48: 1517- 1521.

8) Tang MX, Jacobs D, Stern Y et al. Effect of estrogen during menopause on risk and age at onset of Alzheimer's disease. *Lancet* 1996; 348 (9025): 249- 32.

9) Paganini- Hill A, Henderson VW. Estrogen replacement therapy and risk of Alzheimer's disease. *Arch Intern Med* 1996; 156 (19): 2213- 7.

10) Henderson VW, Watt L, Buckwalter JG. Cognitive skills associated with estrogen replacement in women with Alzheimer's disease. *Psychoneuroendocrinology* 1996; 21 (4): 421- 30.

11) Ohkura T, Isse K, Akazawa K et al. Evaluation of estrogen treatment in female patients with dementia of the Alzheimer's type. *Endocrinology Journal* 1994; 41 (4): 361- 71.

Chapter 5

1) Williams, M.E. In: *The American Geriatrics Society's Complete Guide to Aging and Mental Health*. New York, Random House, Inc., 1995.

2) Walz, T. H., & Blum, N. S. In: *Sexual Health in Later Life*. Lexington, Massachusetts: Lexington Books, 1987.

3) Breecher, E. M. In: *Love, Sex, and Aging*. Boston, MA: Little, Brown and Company, 1984.

4) Crooks, R. & Baur, K. In: *Our Sexuality*. Pacific Grove, CA: Brooks and Cole Publishing Company, 1996.

5) Hodson, D. S., & Skeen, Sexuality and aging: The hammerlock of myths. *The Journal of Applied Gerontology*,1994; (13): 219-235.

6) Kaplan, H. S. (1990). Sex, intimacy, and the aging process. *Journal of the American Academy of Psychoanalysis* 1990; (18): 185-205.

7) Mooradian, A. D.. Geriatric sexuality and chronic diseases. *Clinics in Geriatric Medicine* 1991(7): 113-131.

8) Thienhaus, O. J. Practical overview of sexual function and advancing age. *Geriatrics* 1988(43): 63-67.

Chapter 6

1) Davidson JM, Kwan M, Greenleaf WJ. Hormonal replacement and sexuality in men. *Clin Endocrinol Metab* 1982; 11(3): 599-623.

2) Kwan M, Greenleaf WJ, MannJ et al. The nature of androgen action on male sexuality: a combined laboratory self report study

on hypogonadal men. *J Clin Endocrinol Metab* 1983: 57(3): 557-62.

3) Johnson AR, Jarrow JP. Is routine endocrine testing of impotent men necessary? *J Urol* 1992; 147(6); 1542- 3.

40 Clopper RR, Voorhess Ml, MacGillivray MH et al. Psychosexual behavior in hypopituitary men: a controlled comparison of gonadotrophin and testosterone replacement. *Psychoneuroendocrinology* 1993; 18(2): 149- 61.

5) Sadowsky M, Antonovsky H, Sobel R et al. Sexual activity and sex hormone levels in aging men. *Int Psychogeriatr* 1993; 5(2): 181- 6.

6) Araujo AB, Durante R, Feldman HA et al. The relationship between depressive symptoms and male erectile dysfunction: cross sectional results from the Massachusetts Male Aging Study. *Psychsom Med* 1998; 60(4): 458- 65.

7) Emmanuele AJ, Emiliano S, Eleonora C et al. Lack of sexual activity from erectile dysfunction is associated with a reversible reduction in serum testosterone. *Int J of Andrology* 1999; 22(6); 385- 392.

8) Buvat J, Lemaire A. Endocrine screening in 1022 men with erectile dysfunction: clinical significance and cost effective strategy. *J Urol* 1997: 158(5): 1764- 7.

9) Lue TF. Erectile Dysfunction. *New Eng J Medicine* 2000; 342(24): 1802- 1813.

10) Miller TA. Diagnostic Evaluation of Erectile Dysfunction. *American Family Physician* 2000; 61(1): 95-104.

11) Educational Advances in Sexual Dysfunction; *Postgraduate Medicine* May 2000 Supplement.

Chapter 7

1) Tan RS, Bransgrove LB. Andropause: Is there a role for hormone replacement therapy? *Clinical Geriatrics* 1997; 5(10): 46-58.
2) Tan RS, Bransgrove L: Testosterone replacement therapy - What is its potential in elderly men?
Postgraduate Medicine 103(5):247-256, 1998.
3) Tan RS. Managing the Andropause in aging males. *Clinical Geriatrics* 7(8): 63- 67, 1999.
4) Wang C, Swerdloff RS, Iranmesh A et al. Transdermal testosterone gel improves sexual function, mood, muscle strength and body composition parameters in hypogonadal men. *J Clin Endocrinol Metab* 2000; 85:2839-2853.
5) Cunningham GR, Hirshkowitz M, Korenman SG et al. Testosterone replacement and sleep-related erections in hypogonadal men. *J Clin Endocrinol Metab* 1990; 70(3):792-7.
6) Morley JE, Perry HM. Androgen deficiency in aging men. *Med Clin North Am* 1999; 1279-1289.

Chapter 8

1) Savine R, Sonksen PH. Is the Somatopause an indication for Growth Hormone? *J Endocrinol Invest* 1999: 22:142- 9.
2) Rudman D, Feller AG, Nagraj HS et al. Effects of Human Growth Hormone in men over 60 years old. *New Eng J Medicine* 1990; 323(1); 1-6

3) Rudman D, Shetty KR. Unanswered questions concerning the treatment of hyposomatotropism and hypogonadism in elderly men. *J American Geriatrics Soc* 1994; 42(5): 522-7.

4) Cohn L, Feller AG, Draper MW et al. Carpal Tunnel Syndrome and Gynaecomastia during Growth Hormone treatment of Elderly Men with low circulating IGF-I concentrations. *Clin Endocrinol* 1993: 39(4): 417-25.

5) Gupta KL, Shetty KR, Agre JC et al. Human Growth Hormone effect on serum IGF-I and muscle function in poliomyelitis survivors. *Arch Phys Med Rehab* 1994; 75(8):889-94.

Chapter 9

The web site that you can access further information and purchase supplements on line   www.planetrx.com

Chapter 10

1) Ham RJ, Sloane PD In*: Primary Care Geriatrics*, 2nd ed., St. Louis, Mosby, 1992.

2) Jenike M. In: *Geriatric Psychiatry & Psychopharmacology*, New Haven, Year Book Publishers 1987.

3) Dr. Atkins Diet Revolution. *Med Lett Drugs Ther* 1973; 15(10): 41-42.

4) The web site of the *National Institute of Health*, www.nih.gov will link you to many educational programs on smoking cessation, help for alcoholism and preventive medicine issues.

Index